"Nancy Mohrbacher's *Breastfeeding Solutions* is a handy guide for solving common breastfeeding problems. *Breastfeeding Solutions* is formatted so that new mothers can find the information they need right away, and Mohrbacher offers more than one solution for each problem she describes. That is an important feature, as so many of these problems are complex and the solution may not be readily apparent. When mothers are presented with several ways to address a problem, they more likely to persist until the breastfeeding problem is solved. Mothers will also be encouraged by Mohrbacher's underlying optimism and her firm belief that breastfeeding problems can be solved. This book is a useful guide for both mothers and the practitioners that care for them. I highly recommend it."

> —Kathleen Kendall-Tackett, PhD, IBCLC, FAPA, editor-in-chief of *Clinical Lactation*, coauthor of *Breastfeeding Made Simple*, and owner of Praeclarus Press

"It's always been my impression that breastfeeding gently nudges us into becoming the kind of mother our baby needs. So when problems arise, the clear and effective strategies presented in *Breastfeeding Solutions* are key to getting back on track for a life-enriching breastfeeding experience."

> —Marian Tompson, cofounder of La Leche League International, founder and CEO of AnotherLook, and author of *Passionate Journey: My Unexpected Life*.

D0190645

"Is there room for another breastfeeding book? My enthusiastic answer is, 'yes!' *Breastfeeding Solutions* is a short primer written for busy nursing mothers seeking the latest cutting-edge answers to their concerns in a short and easy format. Nancy Mohrbacher has a way with capsulizing information into concepts like 'The Magic Number' that help mothers understand what is happening and how to fix it, if there really is a problem. If her many solutions don't solve the problem (and they usually will), the excellent resource list will quickly direct mothers to further information on their issue. I will be sending this book to my daughter and daughter-in-law!"

—Lisa Marasco, MA, IBCLC, FILCA, La Leche League Leader, coauthor of *The Breastfeeding Mother's Guide to Making More Milk*

Quick Tips for the Most
Common Nursing Challenges

BREASTFEEDING
SOLUTIONS

NANCY MOHRBACHER
IBCLC, FILCA

New Harbinger Publications, Inc.

Publisher's Note

This publication is designed to provide accurate and authoritative information in regard to the subject matter covered. It is sold with the understanding that the publisher is not engaged in rendering psychological, financial, legal, or other professional services. If expert assistance or counseling is needed, the services of a competent professional should be sought.

Distributed in Canada by Raincoast Books

Copyright © 2013 by Nancy Mohrbacher
New Harbinger Publications, Inc.
5674 Shattuck Avenue
Oakland, CA 94609
www.newharbinger.com

Cover design by Amy Shoup
Acquired by Tesilya Hanauer
Edited by Marisa Solis

Library of Congress Cataloging in Publication Data on file

Printed in the United States of America

15   14   13

10   9   8   7   6   5   4   3   2   1   First printing

Contents

Introduction

Caring for a newborn is a 24/7 labor of love. With a baby in your life, even fitting in a quick shower can sometimes be tricky, so wading through a thick book to find the breastfeeding fix you need is a time-consuming frustration most mothers would rather avoid. This slim volume was written to simplify your life by cutting to the chase. A quick read, it features line drawings, bulleted lists, charts, and other visuals for fast, easy access to the best and most current breastfeeding strategies. It is also organized so that you can skip straight to your burning issue without having to read earlier chapters first.

Why do you need solutions to breastfeeding problems? After all, we're mammals, so shouldn't breastfeeding come naturally? On one level, that makes sense, but unlike other mammals, human mothers have large brains and they can overthink breastfeeding, especially when bombarded with conflicting advice. Plus, many of us grew up with bottlefeeding as the norm, so we try (either consciously or unconsciously) to apply what we know about bottlefeeding to breastfeeding, which often leads to more problems.

Why is solving breastfeeding problems important? The U.S. government commissioned a team of scientists, led by Stanley Ip, who examined existing breastfeeding research and concluded in their 2007 summary that, during the first year of life, babies fed nonhuman milks have more cases of pneumonia, bronchitis, diarrhea, ear infections (up to four times more), urinary tract infections, meningitis, and sudden infant death syndrome (SIDS).

But it's not just about babies. Breastfeeding is also important to moms. In recent years, U.S. physician Alison Stuebe and her colleagues have made the effects of breastfeeding on women's health a major focus of their research. They found that when breastfeeding fails, it increases our risk of the number-one killer of women: cardiovascular disease. Breast and ovarian cancers, metabolic syndrome, type 2 diabetes, and many other life-threatening health problems are also more likely when mothers don't breastfeed or when they wean early. Even decades later, breastfeeding failure has significant negative effects on women's health. Our health care system and economy are also affected. In a 2010 cost analysis published in *Pediatrics*, Melissa Bartick and Arnold Reinhold concluded that if 90 percent of mothers exclusively breastfed for six months, each year this would save $13 billion in U.S. health care costs and prevent 910 infant deaths.

Knowing the importance of breastfeeding, why should you take my advice? Let me share a little about myself: I've been helping breastfeeding families since 1982, first as a volunteer breastfeeding counselor—before lactation as a profession even existed—then, after 1991, as a board-certified lactation consultant. For ten years I worked one on one with thousands of families as the owner of a large private lactation practice in the

Chicago area. The breastfeeding books I've written are used internationally by professionals and parents, and in preparation for writing them, I steeped myself in the latest research and thinking in the field. (For more about me and my books, see my website: www.NancyMohrbacher.com.) One of my books for parents is *Breastfeeding Made Simple: Seven Natural Laws for Nursing Mothers*, which I coauthored with Kathleen Kendall-Tackett, PhD, IBCLC, to provide a clear understanding of basic breastfeeding dynamics.

Think of this book as a companion to *Breastfeeding Made Simple*. Rather than focusing on breastfeeding's seven natural laws, the focus of this book is the practical and often surprising solutions to the seven most common breastfeeding challenges: Latching struggles, worries about milk supply, and nipple and breast pain are the top four. Night feedings, milk expression, and weaning make up the other major concerns.

During my nearly three decades in the breastfeeding field, the prevalence of these seven challenges among mothers has changed very little. But thanks to insights gained from recent research, a *lot* has changed in what lactation professionals know about these issues and how we advise mothers to overcome them.

If you find yourself facing any of these difficulties, my hope is that the suggestions in this book will help you overcome them quickly. Often all it takes is a simple tweak to transform what seems like an insolvable situation into happy and satisfying breastfeeding. But because no book can solve all breastfeeding problems, if, after trying these suggestions, you are still struggling, each chapter describes other, less common possibilities you can pursue with your local breastfeeding support person. If you're not sure where to find skilled, in-person breastfeeding help in your area, see the Resources section at the end of this book.

May this book help you meet your breastfeeding goals!

—Nancy Mohrbacher, IBCLC, FILCA
  Chicago suburbs
  September 2012

Chapter 1

Latching Struggles

Few challenges are more upsetting to both mother and baby than latching struggles. Many mothers whose babies resist taking the breast simply give up in despair. But thanks to more research on this issue, we have new strategies that can help you achieve settled breastfeeding, even when your baby seems to be fighting the breast.

Problem 1: Your newborn or young infant has trouble latching.

Just like other mammal newborns, our babies have inborn reflexes that—when conditions are right—make it possible for them to get to the breast without help. Knowing a little about your baby's reflexes and how gravity affects them can eliminate many wrestling matches at the breast.

Try Laid-Back Breastfeeding

Newborns have at least twenty different reflexes that help them locate the breast, make their way there, latch on, and

Myth: Some babies just don't like breastfeeding.

Reality: Babies are hardwired to breastfeed. Until infant formulas became commercially available, there was no safe substitute for breastfeeding, which makes it a necessary survival skill. If you're having trouble latching, it's not that your baby doesn't like breastfeeding; you just need to find out what the problem is and what adjustment to make.

feed. Thankfully, these reflexes work best when you're in a well-supported and comfortable position.

Until recently, nearly every breastfeeding class taught mothers-to-be the names of specific breastfeeding holds, which they practiced with dolls. But we've discovered that these holds, most of which involve sitting up straight, can actually complicate early breastfeeding.

Why is sitting up straight a problem? After giving birth vaginally, this puts pressure on a very tender area, which can be uncomfortable for you. Also, when you sit up to breastfeed, gravity pulls your baby down and away from you. To orient himself to the breast, your baby needs to have his entire front—face, torso, arms, legs, feet—touching you. Any gaps between you and him can lead to disorientation and frustration. And to keep baby pressed against you at breast height while sitting up straight, you must either find a pillow to support baby's weight that's just the right thickness (not easy) or hold your baby in your arms for long stretches, which can be tiring.

But there's more. When you sit upright, the effects of gravity on your baby's inborn reflexes can make latching difficult. When sitting up or lying on your side, baby's arms may flail and his legs may kick. Head-bobbing may push him away from your breast and his body may arch.

Although some mothers think these movements are signs that their baby doesn't want to breastfeed, nothing could be further from the truth! These are your baby's feeding reflexes in action—but in upright or side-lying positions, gravity turns these same reflexes into major hurdles to feeding. Baby wants to latch, but he's fighting gravity to do so and likely getting frustrated in the process.

Many mothers complain that in upright or side-lying positions they don't have enough hands to contain their babies' hands and feet *and* help them to the breast. If during these struggles baby attaches to the breast at all, he often takes the breast shallowly, which can cause pain for you and frustration for him. A deep latch, on the other hand, triggers his active suckling and makes breastfeeding more comfortable for you. A deeper mouthful of breast also gives baby more milk with every suck.

Leaning back to breastfeed, as researcher Suzanne Colson (who coined the term "laid-back breastfeeding") discovered, can short-circuit many breastfeeding battles. This works because gravity keeps you and your baby in full frontal contact without a lot of effort on your part. Also, gravity works with your baby's reflexes to help him get on the breast deeply, which triggers active suckling and helps him settle quickly.

Tip: When using laid-back, or semi-reclined, feeding positions, you should lean back far enough so that your baby's body can rest comfortably tummy down on top of you but upright enough so that you can see him easily without straining your neck.

While leaning back, make sure your head, neck, shoulders, arms, and legs are all well supported. Think about how you sit or lie back at home when you watch a movie or a television show. If we know we'll be in one position for a long while, we usually find a way to relax all of our muscles. We may scoot our hips forward on a sofa and lean back. We may push back our recliner. We may use pillows in bed to support our head, neck, shoulders, arms, or legs. To see one mother in action in a laid-back breastfeeding position, watch the online video clip at: www.biologicalnurturing.com/video/bn3clip.html. When you breastfeed this way, you can relax completely for as long as your baby feeds, which makes breastfeeding a lot less work.

In semi-reclined feeding positions, gravity works in harmony with your baby's reflexes so that they work the way nature intended. The only way newborns can crawl to the breast after birth without help is if their mother lies back. With gravity helping, the baby's arm and leg movements don't add to your breastfeeding challenges; instead, they move baby toward the breast. His head-bobbing doesn't push him away from your body; instead it raises his head just high enough to hover over your nipple. As baby's head drops to take the breast, gravity pulls it down automatically for a deep latch. When semi-reclined, you don't have to work as hard to make sure baby takes the breast deeply—and most likely your nipples will feel the difference in comfort.

In laid-back positions, you never have to be concerned about whether you're getting it "right." No two mothers and babies are alike, so there's no need to imitate the way someone else breast-feeds. Experiment to find the semi-reclined positions that work best for you. Think of you and your baby as two puzzle pieces. While experimenting, use the following simple adjustments to help you find your best variations:

1. **Adjust how far you're leaning back.** Experiment until you find an angle that works for you. Some mothers prefer a 45-degree angle, while others like their head and shoulders higher or lower.

2. **Adjust the direction your baby lies on your body.** Put baby lengthwise, diagonally, or across your torso until you find a position he likes.

These two dynamics will help you find your own best fit in a variety of breastfeeding positions. If you've had a cesarean, don't worry! Your baby doesn't have to rest on your incision. Figure 1-1 shows several comfortable directions your baby can lie on your body while you're semi-reclined. If you've delivered vaginally, the below-your-breast position and its many variations may work well. If you've had a cesarean, consider the other three positions to avoid putting pressure on your incision during feedings. But these are not your only choices. You have many, many laid-back positions from which to choose.

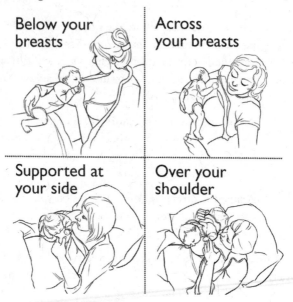

Below your breasts

Across your breasts

Supported at your side

Over your shoulder

Figure 1-1. In laid-back feeding positions, baby can achieve a deeper latch with the help of gravity.

©2012 Anna Mohrbacher, used with permission, adapted from the DVD **Biological Nurturing: Laid-back Breastfeeing** by Suzanne Colson.

Tip: In whatever position you use, make sure that your baby's feet are touching you or something soft near you. Foot contact triggers some of baby's feeding reflexes and, if missing, can contribute to latching struggles. If your baby's feet are sticking out into thin air, adjust his body so that they are touching something soft, such as your body, soft bedding, a couch cushion, or something similar.

Also, although your baby can get to the breast without help in a semi-reclined feeding position, he doesn't have to. Follow your instincts and help him take the breast in any way that feels right to you. For instance, if his nose seems blocked after getting a deep latch, you can make an airway for him by pressing down on the breast with your fingers.

Use Your Baby's Reflexes While Sitting Up or Side-Lying

Laid-back positions are usually easier, especially during your baby's early weeks, but that's not true for everyone. Some mothers prefer to breastfeed sitting up or lying down, at least some of the time, and others find that breastfeeding goes more smoothly in upright or side-lying positions. To accomplish this with the fewest breastfeeding scuffles, understanding how to make your baby's feeding reflexes work for you in these positions is key. It is trickier for baby to take the breast deeply with gravity pulling him down and away from you, but you can help your baby get a deep mouthful of breast by offsetting the effects of gravity.

1. Position baby under your breasts with his whole body (including his hips, legs, and feet) facing and touching you. Make sure there are no gaps between you and him, and that his body is not twisted or turned.

2. Use firm but gentle pressure against baby's shoulders to snuggle his entire body in close. (If lying down, you can wedge a rolled-up towel or baby blanket behind his back with his head free to tilt back.)

3. Align baby's nose (not his lips) to your nipple.

4. Pull baby in closer so that his chin touches the breast. Use a light, steady touch or repeated gentle tapping, which should trigger a wide-open mouth.

5. When his mouth is open wide, help him further onto the breast with gentle pressure behind his shoulders so that he takes the breast deeply, with his lower lip as far from the nipple as possible.

6. Once he's on the breast, make sure his head is free to tilt back slightly for easier swallowing.

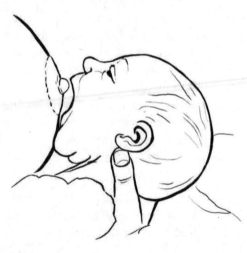

Figure 1-2. Avoid pushing on the back of baby's head when encouraging him to take a deep latch. If you are sitting up, support his head along your forearm or with your palm on baby's back and thumb and forefinger behind baby's ears.

©2012 Anna Mohrbacher, used with permission.

Use the Breast Sandwich or Nipple Tilting for a Deeper Latch

Breast shaping is one way to help a struggling baby get on the breast deeper, which triggers active suckling and helps him settle quickly. It can be used while in a laid-back or any other position. Two popular breast-shaping techniques are the *breast sandwich* and *nipple tilting.*

Breast Sandwich

The breast sandwich can help your baby, at any age, take the breast deeply. But it can be especially useful during the early weeks while you and your baby are learning to breastfeed. It's also a good technique to use when your breasts are firm, which can contribute to latching challenges. In your baby's early days, your breasts may feel harder than usual from engorgement. Later on, they may be firm after missing a feeding. Or your breasts may be naturally firm.

To use the breast sandwich:

1. Gently squeeze your breast near the *areola* (the darker circle around your nipple) to make it narrower, with fingers on one side and thumb opposite.

2. Compress the breast into an oval shape, with the oval of your squeezed breast running in the same direction as the oval of the baby's mouth, making it narrower between his upper and lower lips (figure 1-3). If your baby is lying lengthwise on your body, your fingers and thumb will be in the shape of a "C." If baby's lying at

right angles to your body, your fingers and thumb will be in the shape of a "U."

3. Trigger your baby's wide-open mouth by pulling baby in close—with his entire body touching yours and his chin touching the breast—and using either a light, steady touch or repeated gentle tapping.

4. Once he has opened wide, help baby onto the breast deeply with a gentle push from behind his shoulders.

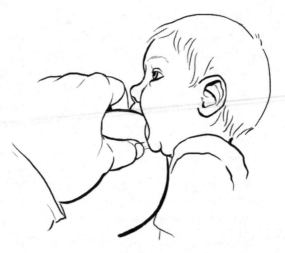

Figure 1-3. Breast sandwich: Gently squeeze the breast so that it is narrower between baby's upper and lower lips for an easier latch.

©2012 Anna Mohrbacher, used with permission.

When you gently compress the breast, make sure that your fingers or thumb are positioned running parallel to baby's lips. And be sure to keep your fingers far enough back on the breast so that they don't get in baby's way as he latches on.

Nipple Tilting

Another way to help baby take a deeper mouthful of breast, nipple tilting involves rolling the underside of the breast into baby's mouth. To do this:

1. Hold your baby close to you with his body against yours and his chin touching the breast.

2. Press into your breast just above the nipple with your thumb running parallel to baby's lips, and point the nipple up and away from baby (figure 1-4).

3. The touch of the breast on your baby's chin should trigger a wide-open mouth.

4. With baby's chin still in contact with the breast, press your thumb into the breast to roll the underside of the breast into baby's wide-open mouth.

5. As the breast enters baby's mouth, use your thumb to gently push the nipple inside baby's upper gum before removing your finger.

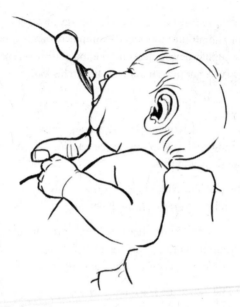

Figure 1-4. Nipple tilting: Roll the nipple into baby's mouth for a deeper latch.

©2012 Anna Mohrbacher

Use Reverse-Pressure Softening If Your Breasts Feel Firm

When the dark circle around your nipple (areola) feels firm rather than soft, this can lead to a latching struggle or a shallow latch, which can mean nipple pain for you and less milk for your baby. *Reverse-pressure softening* (RPS) is an easy way to avoid these problems by making the areola very supple right before feedings. RPS requires no special equipment—just your hands.

RPS should never cause discomfort and should not be used if you have a lump or hardened area in your breast from the painful breast condition known as *mastitis* (see Problem 13 in chapter 4). To do RPS follow these tips:

- Look at figures 1-5 to 1-10 and choose whichever approach seems easiest to you.

- Lie back while doing RPS, so gravity helps move the swelling.

- Gently press inward toward your heart, firmly and steadily, counting slowly to fifty. *Count very slowly if you're very swollen.*

- If you have long fingernails, see figure 1-5 or ask someone else to help (figure 1-9).

- Use RPS to soften the areola right before each feeding or pumping until the swelling goes away.

For some mothers, it may take a few days for the breast swelling to subside. Make any pumping sessions short, with pauses to resoften the area if needed. Use a medium- or low-suction setting on your pump to reduce the return of swelling.

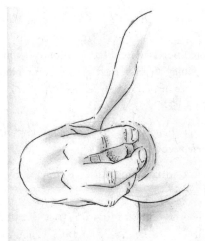

Figure 1-5. One-handed "flower hold": If you have short fingernails, place your curved fingertips where baby's tongue will go. Apply pressure.

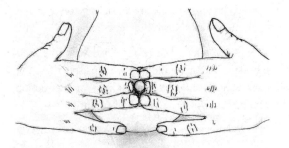

Figure 1-6. Two-handed, one-step method: If you have short fingernails, place hands on the breast so that your curved index, middle, and ring fingertips are touching the nipple. Apply pressure.

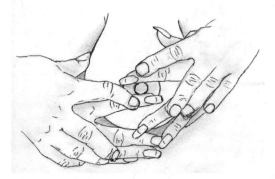

Figure 1-7. If you need assistance, you might ask someone to help press by placing his or her fingers or thumbs on top of yours.

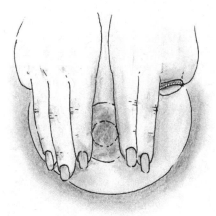

Figure 1-8. Two-step method, two hands: Place two or three straight fingers on each side of the nipple and bend at the knuckles with your remaining fingers. Apply pressure. Move one-quarter turn and repeat until a full circle is made around the nipple.

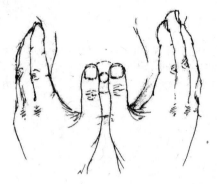

Figure 1-9. Two-step method, two hands: Use straight thumbs on the areola so that the bases of the thumbnails align with the nipple. Apply pressure. Move one-quarter turn and repeat until a full circle is made around the nipple.

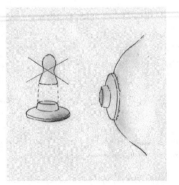

Figure 1-10. Soft-ring method: Cut off the bottom half of an artificial nipple and place it on the areola. Apply pressure with fingers.

Illustrations ©2012 Kyle Cotterman, used with permission. Reverse-pressure softening technique by K. Jean Cotterman, RNC-E, IBCLC.

If These Strategies Don't Work

If the strategies in this section don't lead to settled breast-feeding, don't despair. When a newborn or young infant has trouble latching, there must be a reason. If you can't solve this problem on your own, it's time to get skilled breastfeeding help. See the Resources section to make sense of the various breastfeeding credentials and to find a breastfeeding caregiver with the expertise you need in your area.

If your baby has never breastfed well, your struggles may be related to one or more of the rare situations listed below. This list may help you rule in or out some possible causes of latching problems. Some of these may stem from the baby and some from the mother.

Baby Issues

Baby issues fall into three general categories: anatomy, prematurity, and health.

Anatomy

Most anatomy issues concern baby's mouth and tongue, but some involve baby's breathing. When given a choice, breathing always comes before eating.

- **Is baby tongue-tied?** Is the frenulum (the string-like membrane below the tongue) short enough to prevent normal tongue movement?

- **Does baby have an unusual palate?** The roof of baby's mouth may have an unusual shape or an opening (cleft) in its hard or soft areas or even under the skin (submucosal).

- **Is baby having trouble breathing while breastfeeding?** Some babies are born with breathing problems. If baby has to choose between breathing and eating, breathing always wins!

- **Is baby's upper lip curled under while breastfeeding?** Is the membrane connecting baby's upper lip and gums so tight that baby's upper lip can't flange back?

Prematurity

Many premature babies can breastfeed effectively, especially if they get lots of practice time at the breast. In some cases, though, they're not quite ready to exclusively breastfeed.

- **Was baby born very early?** Some preterm babies may not have the coordination yet to breastfeed well.

- **Has baby been given lots of practice time at the breast?** Practice is even more important than gestational age in preemies' breastfeeding effectiveness.

Health

If a baby is ill or has neurological problems, breastfeeding may take some time and practice to work well.

- **Has baby been diagnosed with neurological problems?** For instance, Down syndrome or any other syndrome?

- **Is baby ill?**

Mother Issues

If your anatomy, health, or low milk production contribute to latching problems, these challenges can usually be overcome with time and skilled breastfeeding help.

Anatomy

Problems related to the nipple and breast are discussed in chapters 3 and 4 respectively. Ask yourself:

- **Is your breast tissue firm or taut?**
- **Do you have flat, inverted, or unusual-shaped nipples?**
- **Are you large-breasted?**
- **Can you express milk?**

Milk Production

If you believe you have low milk production, see chapter 2 for common challenges. Ask yourself:

- **Are you producing ample milk to meet your baby's needs?**
- **Are you producing much more milk than your baby needs?**

Health

Sometimes factors unrelated to breastfeeding contribute to latching problems.

- **Are you ill?**

- **Are you taking any medications, including birth control pills, which may affect milk production?**

Your breastfeeding caregiver can likely help you rule in or out some of these causes for easier problem solving and discuss possible next steps. Remember, babies are hardwired to breast-feed, and if there is a latching problem, there's always a reason.

Problem 2: Baby will only take one breast.

Some babies prefer one breast over the other. If you have a newborn that is taking only one breast, the most common reasons for this are:

- One nipple protrudes more, making it easier to grasp.

- One nipple is easier to manage due to a difference in size or texture.

- One breast is easier to manage because it's less full or less firm.

If your nipple shape, size, or texture is the problem, don't panic! Your newborn or young baby will have an easier time latching within a few days or weeks. Babies' mouths grow very quickly, and their coordination improves as they mature, which makes latching easier.

If you have *mastitis* (also known as a plugged duct or breast infection; see Problem 13), this may cause a baby of any age to refuse one breast. This sometimes happens because mastitis can change the taste of the milk and the milk flow. With mastitis, you'll feel breast pain or tenderness in the affected breast. Any time a baby who was breastfeeding well on both breasts suddenly refuses one breast, see your health care provider to rule out a breast-related medical cause.

Sometimes the reason a baby prefers one breast over the other may not be obvious. Keep in mind that babies can get enough milk by exclusively breastfeeding from one breast. (Moms have exclusively breastfed twins, triplets, even quadruplets!) But most mothers would prefer to use both breasts so that their breasts aren't temporarily lopsided in size. If you want your baby to take both breasts, these strategies may help.

Express Milk from the Unused Breast

Safeguard your milk production in the unused breast by expressing milk at least eight times per day if your baby is less than one month old or at least six times per day if she is older. This will help even out your milk production, which will make the transition to taking both breasts easier for your baby.

Adjust Your Position and When and Where You Breastfeed

To rule out a basic latching problem, first read over the recommendations outlined earlier in this chapter: Use semi-reclined breastfeeding positions, work with baby's reflexes, try a *breast sandwich* or *nipple tilting*, incorporate *reverse-pressure softening*. If baby is still refusing one breast, here are some more suggestions.

- Try a position that allows you to use your dominant hand to help your baby latch.

- Try offering the refused breast when baby is in a light sleep and less aware.

- For a baby older than a month or two, try breastfeeding in a darkened room or try moving her to the refused breast while walking or rocking to distract her.

Most mothers do not produce milk evenly on both sides, but what matters to the baby is her overall milk intake, not how much milk she gets from each breast. Sometimes big differences in milk production or flow between breasts can affect baby's willingness to latch. If you think this might be the cause, and your baby is resistant to the breast with the slower flow, try stimulating milk flow in that breast with a pump or by hand before offering it. If your baby is resistant to the breast with the faster flow, use a position in which her head is higher than the breast (for example, a laid-back position), so that gravity will give her more control over milk flow.

Try the Slide-Over Position

If your baby still refuses one breast, try the *slide-over position*. This works well if your baby is unable to turn her head easily or feels pain when pressure is applied to some areas. Discomfort when being held can also happen when a baby of any age is sore from an immunization or injury, even a minor one. Start by positioning baby at the breast she'll accept. When you hear baby swallowing, keep her body position exactly the same, her head pointed in the same direction, and simply slide her over to the other breast in this exact same position.

If These Strategies Don't Work

As already mentioned, most babies can get all the milk they need from one breast. In fact, one mom of twins exclusively breastfed both babies from one breast after a mastectomy. So if despite all your efforts your baby will not take the other breast, you can continue breastfeeding from one breast. Even if your breasts look lopsided now, that won't be permanent! After your baby weans, your breasts should return to the same size that they were before.

Problem 3: Your baby suddenly refuses the breast.

Have you ever heard the term *nursing strike*? It describes a baby who suddenly refuses the breast after a month or more of uneventful breastfeeding. Some mothers whose babies go "on strike" wonder if this is their baby's way of weaning. But this is unlikely in a baby younger than one year, because during their first year babies have a physical need for mother's milk. Another clue that a nursing strike is not a natural weaning is that the baby is usually unhappy about it. Typically, a nursing strike lasts two to four days, but it may last as long as ten days. It may require some ingenuity to help baby return to breastfeeding.

First Express Your Milk and Feed the Baby

When a baby refuses the breast completely, focus first on two things:

1. Expressing your milk

2. Feeding the baby

Express Your Milk as Often as Baby Was Breastfeeding

This avoids uncomfortable breast fullness and maintains your milk production. Use whatever milk-expression method works best for you: a breast pump or hand expression. Ideally, if your baby isn't nursing at all, a double electric breast pump will make this process faster and easier, as well as more likely to keep up your milk production (see "Your Newborn Isn't Breastfeeding or Your Milk Supply Needs a Boost" in chapter 6).

Feed Your Baby Your Expressed Milk

How you feed your milk will depend in part on your baby's age. A cup is a good choice for a baby at least six to eight months old, and it does not satisfy baby's sucking urge like a bottle. A baby younger than six to eight months can be fed your milk with a cup, spoon, or even an eyedropper. Most mothers think first of feeding their baby with a bottle, but a feeding method that does not satisfy a baby's sucking urge may end the strike sooner.

Tip: When a baby doesn't have other outlets for his sucking urge, such as a bottle or pacifier, he will be more motivated to go back to the breast. Keep this in mind when choosing a feeding method. If your baby has been taking a pacifier regularly, consider giving it a rest until his "nursing strike" is over and he's back to breastfeeding.

Determine the Cause of the Nursing Strike

Why do babies who nursed well for so long suddenly refuse the breast or begin to struggle with latching? Before choosing a strategy, it can be helpful to determine the cause. The possible causes fall into two main categories.

Physical Causes

- Ear infection, cold, or other illness

- Reflux disease, which makes feedings painful

- Overabundant milk production with a fast, overwhelming flow

- Allergy or sensitivity to a food or drug mother consumed

- Pain when held after an injury, medical procedure, or injection

- Mouth pain from teething, thrush, or a mouth injury

- Reaction to a product such as deodorant, lotion, or laundry detergent

Environmental Causes

- Stress, upset, or overstimulation

- Breastfeeding on a strict schedule, timed feedings, or regular interruptions

- Baby left to cry for long periods

- Major change in routine, like traveling, a household move, or mother returning to work

- Yelling or arguments during breastfeeding

- A strong negative reaction when baby bites

- An unusually long separation from you

Determining the cause of your baby's breast refusal may make it easier to choose an effective strategy. For example, if your baby is "on strike" because of an ear infection, the right medical treatment and tincture of time may be the best solution. Likewise, if your baby isn't feeding because there's been a change in her environment or routine, try to re-create the setting she was used to as much as feasible, and give it time.

It is always stressful when a baby refuses the breast, but the good news is that it is almost always possible to overcome a nursing strike and return to breastfeeding. The following basic approaches are a good place to start to reduce your stress and shorten the strike.

Keep the Breast a Pleasant Place

Avoid making the breast a battleground. If your attempts to breastfeed are stressful for your baby, feed another way and instead give baby lots of happy cuddle time at the breast. While your baby's near the breast, talk, laugh, play, and make eye contact. Show him that time there is emotionally rewarding, and make any feeding time away from the breast emotionally neutral. Whenever possible, hold your sleeping baby against your breast during naptimes, because relaxing at breast during sleep can help shorten the strike.

Spend Time Touching and in Skin-to-Skin Contact

When not feeding, hold your baby skin to skin, with baby's bare torso against your skin, and stay that way as much as possible. This is soothing to both of you, and the hormones released make baby more open to breastfeeding. If it is a chilly day, throw a blanket over both of you. Try taking a bath with your baby, and use a sling or baby carrier to keep him close.

Offer the Breast While Baby Is in a Light Sleep or Is Drowsy

Many babies accept the breast again for the first time while asleep or in a relaxed, sleepy state. Try breastfeeding while baby naps. Use feeding positions baby likes best and experiment, starting first with laid-back positions (see figure 1-1) to make the most of your baby's natural feeding reflexes. Allow your baby to take naps on your breast when you're in a semi-reclined position.

Get the Milk Flowing Right Away

Pump before offering your breast to give baby an instant reward—flowing milk he doesn't have to work for. Also, first try hand-expressing a little milk onto baby's lips. If baby goes to the breast, but won't stay there, ask a helper to drip expressed milk on the breast or in the corner of baby's mouth with a spoon or eyedropper. Swallowing your milk will trigger suckling, which triggers swallowing. If baby comes off the breast, offer more expressed milk and try again.

Try Breast Shaping and Breastfeeding in Motion

Shaping the breast so that it's easier to latch may help baby take the breast deeper and therefore trigger active suckling. See "Use the Breast Sandwich or Nipple Tilting for a Deeper Latch" earlier in this chapter. Keep in mind that some babies accept the breast only while being walked or rocked, so if baby is not responding to laid-back positions, it may be time to get moving.

Try Breastfeeding When Baby's Not Ravenous

To feed well, baby needs to feel calm and open to breastfeeding rather than hungry and stressed. If baby seems agitated, try ways to calm him first, and try shortening the time between feedings. Some babies will take the breast more easily if they are not very hungry, so try feeding a little milk first, using whatever feeding method is working for you. Start with maybe one-third to one-half of his usual feeding, just to take the edge off his hunger before offering the breast.

Breastfeed as Much as Possible When It's Working

When baby begins accepting the breast, breastfeed for as long as baby will suckle. And offer the breast again soon, rather than waiting for a long stretch or until he is very hungry. Make the most of those times that breastfeeding is going well.

Tip: If your baby takes a bottle but not the breast, try a *bait-and-switch*. Start by bottlefeeding in a breastfeeding position and, while baby is actively sucking and swallowing, pull out the bottle nipple and insert yours. Some babies will just keep suckling.

Use Breastfeeding Tools

Trying the following devices, with the guidance of a lactation professional, may help you turn the corner.

- **Silicone nipple shield.** In some cases, nipple shields can help a baby transition back to the breast, especially if the strike followed a period of heavy bottle and pacifier use. Nipple shields are available in most baby stores and online. For two different brands, sizes, and styles, see: www.amedadirect.com/ameda-nipple-shield.html and www.medelabreastfeedingus.com/products/583 /contact-nipple-shields. With a baby younger than one week, try the Medela 20-mm size. For older babies, the 24-mm size will probably be a better fit.

- **At-breast supplementer.** This product provides immediate milk flow at the breast through a thin tube that attaches to a container. If slow milk flow is an issue, this device may help the baby accept the breast and keep breastfeeding. If slow flow is not the issue, it may not be a good choice. See "Try an At-Breast Supplementer" in chapter 2.

If These Strategies Don't Work

If the strategies in this section don't lead to settled breastfeeding, it's time to get skilled breastfeeding help. See the Resources section to find someone in your area. If your "on-strike" baby is older than two or three months of age, your technique may need a simple tweak or you may need some breastfeeding tools or help with how to use them.

Remember, breastfeeding is the biological norm for mothers and babies. Nearly all breastfeeding struggles have a solution. It's just a matter of finding it. Even if settled breastfeeding seems impossible now, with time, patience, and skilled help you can make breastfeeding work again.

Chapter 2

Milk-Supply Issues

The most common reason mothers wean before they'd planned is worries about milk production. These worries are often rooted in misunderstandings about how milk production works and how to know whether baby is getting enough milk. Some mothers really do make too little milk, which can be upsetting and demoralizing, while others have the opposite problem and struggle with overabundant milk. All of these situations—too little milk, too much milk, and just the right amount—are covered in this chapter, along with strategies for keeping up milk production long term when employment separates you and your baby.

Problem 4: Your newborn isn't satisfied for long and sometimes wants to nurse constantly.

With the birth of their first baby, many new parents are unsure about what's in store—and can be shocked by the surprising number of times a newborn wants to nurse. But anxiety can strike even experienced parents when a new baby's breastfeeding pattern is entirely different from their previous experiences.

Learn About Breastfeeding Norms

During the first six weeks or so, breastfed babies often feed unpredictably. This is not what most first-time parents expect. They hear that newborns typically breastfeed eight to twelve times per day (usually true) and they do the math and assume their baby will breastfeed every two to three hours (not usually true). Unfortunately, some health care providers also offer the same misguided advice. As a result, when baby is obviously hungry before two hours have passed, many moms worry that breastfeeding is not working and that they're not making enough milk. But as you'll discover in this section, wanting to breastfeed again soon after feeding is not a sign your milk production is low. More consistent feeding times should not be expected until after your baby reaches about six weeks of age.

Myth: Your newborn will feed every two to three hours.

Reality: An older child will likely have a more consistent nursing pattern that is similar to this. But most babies under six weeks of age will feed erratically, often much sooner than every two hours.

Early Breastfeeding in a Nutshell

What should you expect during the early weeks? Let's start at the beginning. While in the womb, your baby never felt hunger. She was fed constantly by the nutrients flowing through the umbilical cord. After birth, she feels hunger for the first time. Digesting milk in her stomach and experiencing hunger pangs between feedings are new experiences. To make this transition easier, nature starts your baby off gradually, with small, frequent feedings.

From Your Baby's Perspective

Small feedings are better than larger feedings because at birth your newborn's stomach is tiny. An average feeding on baby's first day is about one-third of an ounce (10 mL) of *colostrum*, the early milk waiting and ready in your breasts at baby's birth. Colostrum provides concentrated nutrition in just the right amounts. Each day during the first week of life, as your milk production increases with frequent nursing, your baby consumes more milk per feeding and her stomach expands. By three days of age, her stomach comfortably holds about 1 ounce (30 mL) of milk.

During baby's first six weeks, assuming you breastfeed whenever baby shows signs of hunger—such as rooting, hand-to-mouth, fussing—two important dynamics affect her feeding pattern: baby's stomach size and your milk production. Table 2-1 shows how these two variables normally increase during your baby's first month.

Table 2-1. Baby's Average Feeding Volume by Age

Baby's Age	Average Volume per Feeding	Average Volume per Day
1 day	0.2 oz. (10 mL)	2 oz. (50 mL)
3 days	1 oz. (30 mL)	8 oz. (250 mL)
1 week	1.5 oz. (45 mL)	15 oz. (450 mL)
2 weeks	2 oz. (60 mL)	20 oz. (600 mL)
1 month	3–4 oz. (90–120 mL)	25–30 oz. (750–900 mL)
6 months	3–4 oz. (90–120 mL)	30 oz. (900 mL)

Trying to stretch out your baby's stomach earlier can be done but is not in her best interest. As is recommended for adults, it's healthier for baby to have small, frequent feedings. Scientists have found that a greater-than-normal weight gain during the first week of life is a risk factor for adult obesity. And regular overfeeding establishes an unhealthy eating pattern that can lead to being overweight later.

From Your Perspective

What does all this mean to you? When breastfeeding is going normally, small feedings during the first six weeks often translate to periods of very frequent and sometimes nonstop breastfeeding. Unlike many babies fed by bottle, most breastfed newborns do not feed at regular time intervals. While it is true that most young babies breastfeed eight to twelve times every twenty-four hours, the usual laws of mathematics simply don't apply here.

During the first six weeks or so, your baby probably won't feed on any kind of regular schedule. Most new babies tend to bunch their feedings together at certain times (called *cluster nursing*) and go longer between feedings at other times. If you're lucky, these longer stretches (up to four to five hours is fine) will be at night. But don't get your hopes up. At first these longer stretches will probably be during the day, since most babies are born with their days and nights mixed up.

Your baby wanting to breastfeed soon after a feeding is not a sign that your milk production is low. It's a sign that your baby is doing a good job of bringing in abundant milk. Regular feeding patterns are unusual during the first six weeks.

Why do many babies cluster their feedings in the evening?

A breast is not like a faucet, with the milk at the same level day and night. Your milk has its own natural ebb and flow, which affects your baby's feeding pattern.

During mornings, milk production is usually at its highest. Mothers often report that their babies go longer between feedings in the morning than in the evening, when milk production is at its lowest ebb. To get the milk they need in the evening, babies feed more often, every hour or even every half hour. This is a completely normal pattern and does not mean that your milk production is low.

These evening breastfeeding marathons are usually confined to the first six weeks. With growth, your baby's stomach gets bigger and can hold more milk. And with practice at the breast, baby learns to get more milk more quickly. With time, your breastfeeding pattern will change, usually becoming more predictable. What's important about this for your baby is not the ebb and flow; it's the total amount of milk she gets every twenty-four hours.

Worried about baby getting enough hindmilk?

Some mothers have heard that the fat content of their milk changes during the course of a breastfeeding, which is true. The first milk baby consumes is thinner and lower in fat than the milk she'll get later in the feeding, because fat sticks to your milk-making glands—and the longer baby feeds, the more fat is released into the milk. However, knowing this has created anxiety in many women, who worry about whether their baby is getting "enough" of the fatty *hindmilk*. Thankfully, this is not something you need to be concerned about. Why? The following facts explain:

- **You don't make "two kinds of milk."** There is no magic moment when foremilk becomes hindmilk. As the baby breastfeeds, the increase in fat content is gradual, with the milk becoming fattier and fattier over time as baby drains the breast more fully.

- **The total milk consumed daily—not the hindmilk—determines baby's weight gain.** Whether babies breastfeed often for shorter periods or go for hours between feedings and feed longer, their total daily fat consumption does not actually vary.

- **Foremilk is not always low-fat**. The fat content of the foremilk varies greatly by breastfeeding pattern. For example, if baby breastfeeds again soon after the last feeding, that foremilk may be higher in fat than the hind-milk consumed at other feedings.

The takeaway message here is that there is no reason to worry about how much hindmilk your baby is getting or to coax her to feed longer. As long as baby breastfeeds effectively and you do not regularly cut feedings shorter than baby wants, she will receive about the same amount of milk fat during the course of a day no matter what her breastfeeding pattern. This is because the baby who breastfeeds more often consumes foremilk higher in fat than the baby who breastfeeds less often. So in the end it all evens out.

There's also no reason to focus on how many minutes baby feeds. Just like adults, some babies consume a lot in just a few minutes, while others are slower eaters and take much longer to consume the same amount.

Know That Exclusive Pumping Will Not Save Time

Some mothers are tempted to take control of their baby's feeding pattern and "save time" by giving up on breastfeeding altogether and instead exclusively pumping their milk and bottle-feeding it to their baby. Bottlefeeding expressed milk may mean more-regular feeding intervals during baby's first weeks—but be mindful. Most mothers who have exclusively pumped for their babies long term say that it was ultimately so time-consuming that they could not keep it up for as long as they had planned to breastfeed. For that reason, most say they would never go down that road again.

Myth: Breastfeeding will always be as time-intensive as it is from day one.

Reality: By six weeks, baby's stomach has grown bigger and can hold more milk. With practice, baby breastfeeds faster and needs fewer feedings each day. After six weeks, breastfeeding usually takes much less time than the alternative: pumping. If you devote the initial extra time to breastfeeding after birth, it ultimately becomes a huge time-saver.

As the months pass, exclusive pumping ultimately takes far more time and work than breastfeeding. Some estimate it takes two to three times longer than breastfeeding because at each feeding mothers do triple duty: first pump, then feed, and then clean their pump equipment and feeding gear.

Think of these early weeks of intensive breastfeeding as an investment that pays back many times over as your baby grows. If you stick with it, as baby's stomach grows and she takes more milk more quickly, breastfeeding increasingly takes less and less time. In fact, by about six weeks or so, many moms find that breastfeeding takes less time than bottlefeeding, even bottlefeeding formula. Getting in sync with your baby's feeding rhythm now will ultimately save you much more time later and build a healthy milk supply in the process.

Problem 5: Your baby is not gaining enough weight.

Being told your baby's weight gain is too low can be a real emotional blow. But before assuming you need to increase milk production, first ask some questions.

Find Out Which Growth Chart Was Used

Is baby's place on the growth chart the concern? If so, first ask if your health care provider is using the growth chart created by the World Health Organization that is based on the growth of exclusively breastfed babies or whether it is based on formula-fed babies. Weight gain norms vary by feeding method.

How is the chart being interpreted? Growth charts can be confusing to both parents and health professionals. A baby's growth is plotted on a series of percentile lines, with an average child at the 50th percentile. This means that out of 100 healthy children, 49 will weigh less and 50 will weigh more.

A weight at a higher percentile is not necessarily "good" and a weight at a lower percentile is not necessarily "bad." By definition, there are thriving children at every percentile. Some will be chunky and some will be petite, but their percentile does not necessarily reflect their health or growth. It is common, for example, for a baby born preterm to be at a low percentile at first, even when he is growing and gaining weight well. On the other hand, a baby may be born at the 95th percentile in weight because of pregnancy-related factors, such as a diabetic mother's high blood-sugar levels or a large pregnancy weight gain, and he may fall in the percentiles as his growth adjusts to his natural norm.

A baby's weight gain throughout weeks and months is what provides an accurate picture of how breastfeeding is going. If a baby is gaining consistently and well, his actual percentile is irrelevant. But if over time his percentile drops, this would be a reason to take a closer look at breastfeeding to see if adjustments are needed.

Compare Your Baby's Weight Gain to the Averages

No matter what else is happening in terms of your baby's feeding patterns, sleep patterns, or fussy times, if you are exclusively breastfeeding and your baby is gaining weight well, your milk production is fine.

Babies typically gain faster during the first three to four months than they will at any other time in their lives. Then their growth slows, which is a good thing. If it didn't, our babies would become giants. Table 2-2 lists average weight gains for breastfeeding babies during their first year.

Table 2-2. Average Weight Gain for Breastfeeding Babies

Age	Weight Gain	
Birth–4 days	Lose up to 7–10% of birth weight	
4 days–4 months	7–8 oz./wk. (200–230 g/wk.)	2 lbs./mo. (0.90 kg/mo.)
4–6 months	4–5 oz./wk. (113–142 g/wk.)	1 lb./mo. (0.45 kg/mo.)
6–12 months	3–4 oz./wk. (85–113 g/wk.)	¾ lb./mo. (0.34 kg/mo.)

Some health care providers tell mothers they "like" babies to gain even more weight than average. But with the current childhood obesity epidemic, this suggestion should be viewed with suspicion.

If, on the other hand, your baby has been losing weight or there is a valid concern about his weight gain, here are some strategies to help boost your milk production.

Learn How Milk Production Works

One of the most important dynamics affecting milk production is how full or drained your breasts are. Known as *degree of breast fullness*, this boils down to a very simple concept: drained breasts make milk faster, and full breasts make milk slower.

Whenever your breasts become full, milk production slows. This happens when the milk begins to exert more pressure in your breasts and there is an increase in the amount of *feedback inhibitor of lactation* (FIL), a substance in the milk. As milk fills your breasts, increasing pressure and FIL sends a signal to your breasts to slow your milk production. The more pressure and FIL in your breasts, the stronger the signal. The fuller your breasts become, the slower you make milk.

The opposite is also true. Milk production speeds when your breasts are drained more fully. That is why a baby who needs more milk feeds more often and longer, taking a larger percentage of the available milk. This is how, during the first month, your newborn increases your milk production to meet his growing needs.

Many mothers assume that babies take all of their available milk at each feeding, but, on average, babies take about two-thirds of the milk in the breasts. This means that at an average feeding one-third of the milk is left.

The bottom line: The more drained your breasts are at the end of a feeding and the more times each day they are well

Myth: Your breasts are empty after your baby nurses.

Reality: On average, most babies take only about two-thirds of your milk. If baby's still hungry, give both breasts more than once. The breasts are continually making milk and are never empty.

drained, the faster you make milk. This concept is the basis for many of the following strategies for boosting milk production.

Breastfeed More

Breastfeed at least eight to twelve times per day, and drain your breasts as fully as possible each time by offering each breast more than once. Go back and forth from breast to breast as many times as baby is willing. Focus on the number of feedings per day, not the time between feedings. Encourage baby to breastfeed whenever he shows feeding cues, such as rooting, hand-to-mouth, or fussing, even if it has only been a short time since he last ate.

If your baby is sleeping so much that breastfeeding at least eight times per day is a challenge, keep in mind that babies can breastfeed very effectively during light sleep. Rather than trying to wake a baby in a deep sleep, which can be an exercise in frustration, lean back into a semi-reclined feeding position (not flat on your back) and lay baby tummy down on your body between your breasts (see figure 1-1). You may need to help him latch.

Get a Deeper Latch

With a bigger mouthful of breast, baby can remove more milk more quickly, which signals your body to increase milk production. Remember: drained breasts make milk faster.

How can you help your baby get a deeper latch? If you're sitting up or lying on your side, this involves making sure baby's body is pressed against yours (no gaps) and bringing his chin into contact with your breast, either with a light, soft touch or a tapping movement. Once he opens wide, apply gentle pressure from behind his shoulders as he latches to gently push the breast deeper into his mouth. See "Use Your Baby's Reflexes While Sitting Up or Side-Lying" and figure 1-2 for more tips on getting a deeper latch.

One easier (and to some surprising) way to get a deeper latch is to use laid-back, or semi-reclined, feeding positions, which use gravity to help baby get farther onto the breast. Many are not familiar with this approach, because the sitting-up and side-lying breastfeeding positions have been recommended for so long.

To get into a laid-back position, lean back far enough so that baby can lie supported tummy down on your body but upright enough that you can see him easily without straining your neck (see figure 1-1 for examples). When you place baby tummy down between your exposed breasts, baby's inborn feeding behaviors are triggered and he may bob his way to the breast. If he seems to need your help, feel free, but you don't need to worry about aligning him in any particular way. See "Try Laid-Back Breastfeeding" in chapter 1 for complete directions.

Use Breast Compression

Breast compression, which was popularized by Canadian pediatrician Jack Newman, MD, can teach a baby who spends a lot of time "at the bar but not drinking" to stay active at the breast. It is usually needed for a few days at most if done consistently at every feeding.

When using breast compression, leave your baby on the first breast to "finish" before switching. You'll know baby is finished when he no longer uses the type of suck in which he opens his mouth wide, pauses, and closes his mouth. He may look like he's just "nibbling."

To do breast compression:

1. If you're in a sitting position, hold the baby with one arm and hold your breast with the opposite hand. If you're laid back, hold your breast with a free hand.

2. Position your thumb on one side of the breast and your other fingers on the other, well away from the nipple and the areola, the dark circle around your nipple.

3. Watch for the wide jaw movements that tell you your baby is getting milk. The baby gets more milk when he is drinking with an open mouth wide–pause–close mouth type of suck. (Open mouth wide–pause–close mouth is one suck; the pause is not a pause between sucks.)

4. When baby is nibbling or no longer drinking with the open mouth wide–pause–close mouth type of suck, compress the breast. Not so hard that it hurts, and try not to change the shape of the breast near baby's mouth. With the compression, baby should start drinking again with the open mouth wide–pause–close mouth type of suck.

5. Keep the pressure up (don't stop compressing) until baby is no longer drinking milk actively even with the compression, then release the pressure. Often baby will stop sucking when the pressure is released but will start again shortly as milk starts to flow. If baby does not stop sucking with the release of pressure, wait a short time before compressing again.

6. Release the pressure to allow your hand to rest and to allow milk to start flowing to baby again. The baby, if he stops sucking when you release the pressure, will start again when he starts to taste milk.

7. When baby starts sucking again, he may drink (open mouth wide–pause–close mouth). If not, compress again as above.

8. Continue on the first side until baby does not drink even with the compression. You should allow baby to stay on this side for a short time longer, as you may occasionally get another milk release and baby will start drinking again on his own. If baby no longer drinks, however, allow him to come off or take him off the breast.

9. When breast compression no longer works to keep baby active, break the suction and take him off the breast. Change his diaper or stimulate him by stroking or undressing him more, then offer the other breast. Repeat as many times as needed until baby is done.

Some pauses during breastfeeding are normal. Breast compression is only needed if baby spends much of each nursing session lazing at the breast rather than drinking milk. Breast compression works because it provides an underfeeding baby with positive reinforcement for active suckling. More milk intake promotes more active breastfeeding. In most cases, using breast compression religiously for just a few days is all that is needed, because in that amount of time baby will have learned to stay active without it.

Pump Regularly

Because drained breasts make milk faster, adding regular breast pumping to your day can turn around low milk production and provide your milk as a supplement for the baby who needs more milk right away. The more times per day the breasts are well drained, either by breastfeeding or pumping, the faster milk production increases. Here are some approaches you can try.

- *Double-pump* **(pump both breasts at the same time) for ten to fifteen minutes**, either right after feedings or thirty to sixty minutes later, whichever works better for you. If you wait for a half hour or more, you'll usually get more milk.

- **Pump for an additional two minutes** *after* **you see the last drop of milk**, or for a total of twenty to thirty minutes, whichever comes first, to increase milk production faster.

- **Practice** *hands-on pumping*, which involves massaging your breasts, double-pumping, then single pumping with compression. This technique can boost your milk production by as much as 50 percent. See "Try Hands-On Pumping" in chapter 6 for step-by-step directions.

Hands-on pumping will be easier if you use a hands-free pumping device. Several are available that fit any brand of pump and can be worn over your bra. You can find them by doing an Internet search for "hands-free breast pumping." See also Problem 17.

If your baby is breastfeeding effectively, spend more of your time breastfeeding than pumping. If your baby is ineffective at the breast, focus your time and efforts mainly on pumping until you figure out (with professional assistance) how to help your baby remove more milk while breastfeeding.

Try Taking Fenugreek or Prescription Medications

There are some herbs and prescription medications that can help increase milk supply. But like any supplement, they may interact with drugs you are taking, and should be avoided if you have certain health problems, so discuss them with your health care provider before taking them.

Fenugreek

Taking the herb fenugreek, which is used in artificial maple syrup and in cooking, may increase your milk production. This herb has a long history of international use by breastfeeding mothers, especially in India and Egypt. The U.S. Food and Drug Administration gave fenugreek a rating of Generally Recognized as Safe, but it can interact with a few prescription and over-the-counter medications. You can buy fenugreek at health-food stores and many grocery stores. The dose needed to increase milk production is higher than that recommended on most fenugreek bottles. Take three to four capsules (of at least 500 mg each) three times per day (nine to twelve per day). You know you're taking enough when your sweat and urine smell like maple syrup.

Prescription Medications

Two prescription medications that increase milk production are metoclopramide (Reglan) and domperidone (Motilium). Both drugs are prescribed to relieve certain stomach problems.

Domperidone is currently not recommended for breastfeeding mothers by the FDA, due to side effects reported in very ill individuals receiving domperidone intravenously. However, it is used often to increase milk production in many other countries at its recommended dose of 10 to 40 mg three to four times per day.

Since depression can be a side effect of metoclopramide, avoid it if you have a history of depression. There is also a rare side effect that may occur from using metoclopramide for longer than one month called *tardive dyskinesia*, or involuntary grimacing. These side effects make metoclopramide a less-than-optimal choice. But it can be helpful when used short term in some circumstances. Its recommended dose is 10 to 15 mg three times per day.

Once your milk supply is meeting your baby's needs, gradually taper off of any medications by 10 mg per week for several weeks. It may also be helpful to taper off of herbs gradually rather than stopping them suddenly. This will help minimize a sharp impact on milk production.

Try an At-Breast Supplementer

These devices consist of a container with one or two long, thin tubes that extend into baby's mouth during breastfeeding to provide extra milk at the breast. Advantages of supplementing at breast are:

- Baby is fed once without needing a supplemental feed after breastfeeding.

- Baby stimulates the breast, boosting milk production by taking milk from the breast and simultaneously receiving the supplement from the tube.

- Baby gets positive reinforcement for breastfeeding.

Some mothers are very comfortable using these devices. Others find them difficult to use and clean, and prefer to supplement their babies in other ways. Examples of at-breast supplementers include the Lact-Aid Nursing Trainer, the Medela Supplemental Nursing System (SNS), and the Medela Starter SNS.

If These Strategies Don't Work

When baby's weight gain falters, there are three main factors to consider.

- Baby's breastfeeding effectiveness

- Baby's health

- Your milk production

Any one of these three factors can affect a baby's weight gain. If you have previously breastfed a baby who gained weight normally, you have a "proven breast." Unless you've had breast surgery or an injury, or another health condition has affected milk production, your ability to produce milk is not in question. But even so, if your baby does not breastfeed well and consistently, this will eventually slow your milk production.

What can cause ineffective breastfeeding? One common cause is *tongue-tie*. A baby is considered tongue-tied when the membrane that connects his tongue to the floor of his mouth is so short that it restricts the tongue movements needed for effective milk removal. (See "Tongue-Tie" in chapter 3.) Other anatomical variations, such as an unusual palate (roof of the mouth), can also affect breastfeeding.

A baby born very prematurely will eventually learn to effectively breastfeed, but to get there he will need lots of practice time at the breast. Some infant health conditions can affect breastfeeding, such as Down syndrome, neurological issues, respiratory problems, and cardiac defects. In some rare cases, a breastfeeding baby may actually take enough milk at the breast but gain weight slowly due to a metabolic disorder, a heart defect, or other health condition.

When considering your milk production, keep in mind that until 150 years ago or so, breastfeeding was necessary for the survival of the human race. As a result, milk production tends to be a very hardy process. In fact, some are surprised to learn that even adoptive mothers who have never been pregnant can produce milk for their babies simply by regularly nursing them.

However, as with every other organ in the body, not all breasts function normally. Your anatomy and hormonal health can affect milk production. And as mentioned, reduced milk production (which is reversible with the suggestions in this section) can occur if your baby is not removing milk well from your breasts. If you think your ability to produce milk may be the issue, see an international board-certified lactation consultant (IBCLC), who can troubleshoot with you and review your options. Another excellent resource is the book *The Breastfeeding Mother's Guide to Making More Milk*, by lactation consultants Diana West and Lisa Marasco, which describes in detail what's currently known about all the physical factors that can affect your milk production.

Problem 6: You and your baby struggle with too much milk.

Is it really possible to make too much milk? Definitely! And there are serious drawbacks to overabundant milk production, both for you and your baby.

Drawbacks for you may include uncomfortable breast fullness between feedings and bouts of *mastitis*, a painful breast condition that may include fever and require antibiotic treatment (see Problem 13). Regular and prolonged breast fullness is one of the risk factors for mastitis.

Drawbacks for your baby include overwhelming milk flow and digestive problems. Imagine if someone poured a large volume of liquid into your mouth but gave you no way to control the flow. A baby may try to cope with overabundant milk by pushing away from the breast, pulling back or clamping down on the nipple, or refusing to breastfeed altogether. She may gulp, choke, or sputter when she nurses, and she may seem unusually gassy or have frothy or explosive stools. Some babies cope more easily with overabundant milk over time, as their sucking, swallowing, and breathing become more coordinated.

What should you do if this sounds like you?

Try Positions That Give Baby More Control

With too much milk production, the feeding positions that are most challenging are those in which milk flows downhill into baby's mouth. A good short-term strategy is to try positions that make milk flow easier for your baby to manage. Laid-back breast-feeding positions (see figure 1-1) are ideal, because baby's head is above the breast and gravity slows milk flow. Lying on your side to breastfeed can also help because your baby can let overflow milk dribble out of her mouth (be sure to put down a towel first!), rather than struggling to swallow to keep from choking. Most important is to never hold your baby's head to your breast when she wants to pull off and catch her breath.

Adjusting your feeding position may help baby, but, unfortunately, it won't necessarily help you. Slowing milk production, however, will help both of you. But before taking this step, you need to be certain of one thing first.

Make Sure Too Much Milk Is the Real Problem

Before reducing your milk production, first make sure the problem doesn't have another cause. For example, a baby struggling with milk flow at the breast may have breathing or heart issues. A baby who is gassy or has explosive stools may have a gastrointestinal illness or a food sensitivity. (Gassiness and explosive stools are sometimes associated with very overabundant milk production, because it's difficult for baby to drain each breast fully enough to get to the fatty hindmilk, but this is rare.) One of the easiest ways to confirm overabundant milk is to compare your baby's weight gain to the average.

Tip: A breastfeeding newborn will gain an average of 2 pounds (.90 kg) per month for the first four months. If baby's weight gain is double this or more, overabundant milk production is likely the cause.

Decide If You Want to Slow Your Milk Production

If baby's weight gain is at least twice the average, consider taking steps to slow your milk production. Some mothers struggle with even the idea of doing this. We live in a culture where many consider milk production to be fragile and easily lost. Many mothers worry about reducing their milk for fear they'll end up with the opposite problem: too little milk.

But milk production is a very hardy process. If making less milk will make life better for you and your baby, go ahead. If later you decide that you really hate making less milk, you can always increase your milk production again. The solutions for Problem 5 will show you how.

Use Only One Breast Per Feeding

One of the simplest things you can do to reduce your milk production is to limit each feeding session to only one breast. You can return to that same breast as many times at that feeding as needed if baby still seems hungry. Switch breasts only at the next feeding time, not during a feeding.

If your unused breast starts to feel full before the next feeding, *pump to comfort* on that side, which simply means expressing just enough milk to make you comfortable and no more. You don't want to completely drain that breast or it will signal your body to keep making lots of milk. Using one breast per feeding along with pumping to comfort, if needed, allows your milk production to slow gradually and comfortably without causing pain or increasing health complications.

Does your baby already take only one breast per feeding? This is not uncommon among mothers who make lots of milk. If this describes you, move on to the following solutions.

Try Block Feeding with or without Pumping

Block feeding involves using the same breast for blocks of three hours at a time, along with practicing the pump-to-comfort technique on the other breast as needed until its milk production slows. Baby can feed as often as she likes, but only on the same breast for up to three hours. After that three-hour block ends, offer the other breast for the next three-hour block of time. Continue this cycle until your milk production is more manageable for you and your baby, then go back to your usual feeding pattern, ideally letting the baby nurse as long as she likes on the first breast and then offering the second breast, which she may or may not take.

If this isn't enough to bring your overabundant production under control, you can extend the time blocks to four hours, five hours, or even longer.

To prevent mastitis, also known as plugged ducts or a breast infection (see Problem 13), some suggest using a breast pump to completely drain the breasts on the morning of the first day that you start block feeding. Once milk has been drained from the breasts as completely as possible, put baby immediately to breast. This will begin the first of several three-hour feeding blocks, as described above. As days pass, if your breasts continue to become very full, you can use the breast pump again to drain you fully in the morning. Most mothers, though, only need to drain their breasts with the pump once.

It's important to use block feeding for no more than five to seven days. It is not meant to be a long-term strategy. Your goal is bring down your milk production to a level that is comfortable for you and your baby—not to continue to reduce it after that.

If These Strategies Don't Work

In extreme cases, some herbs and medications can be used to help slow milk production. See your local international board-certified lactation consultant (IBCLC) to discuss using sage, pseudoephedrine, or birth-control pills in this way. You should also get approval from your health care provider, who can ensure that the supplements are okay, given your health history.

Problem 7: Your milk supply is decreasing after returning to work.

Many mothers plan to breastfeed their baby for a minimum of one year, which is recommended by the American Academy of Pediatrics. But when you return to work during this first year, meeting this goal may be tricky.

If returning to work brings with it a gradual slowing of milk production, this section describes a concept—the *magic number*—that explains in part how long-term milk production works and may help you reverse this trend. You'll also find some strategies for pumping more milk at each session, and an explanation for how starting solids impacts milk production. Let's start by calculating how much milk your baby should be taking while you're at work.

Compare Your Baby's Milk Intake with What's Expected

To thrive, most babies between one and six months of age need about 30 ounces (900 mL) of milk per day. Assuming your baby takes milk steadily around the clock, if you and your baby are apart for eight to twelve hours during your workday, your baby will need on average 10 to 15 ounces (300 to 360 mL) of milk. This is one-third of 30 ounces (900 ml) for eight hours and one-half of 30 ounces for twelve hours. If your baby is sleeping the entire night, this means the full 30 ounces will be needed during his daytime hours. More on that later.

While you're at work, if your baby is taking much more milk than expected, consider these possible reasons.

Myth: As they grow, breastfed babies need increasingly more milk per day between one and six months of age.

Reality: This is true for formula-fed babies, but not for breastfed babies, whose milk intake stays remarkably stable between one and six months of age because their rate of growth slows. At around six months, when a breastfed baby starts eating solid foods, his need for mother's milk decreases.

- The bottles contain too much milk and much is being discarded after feedings.

- A fast-flow nipple is used to feed baby, which may cause overfeeding.

- The caregiver is overusing feeding as a way to calm your baby rather than holding or interacting with him.

- Baby needs to compensate for too little breastfeeding while you're together.

If one of the above is the cause, often adjustments can be made to decrease the amount of milk needed while you're away.

Keep an Eye on Your Magic Number

Your magic number is the average number of times your baby breastfed each twenty-four-hour day while you were home on maternity leave. Determining your magic number, however, is based on the following assumptions: that your maternity leave was at least six weeks long; that you were breastfeeding whenever your baby indicated the need, rather than on a fixed time schedule; and that you were exclusively breastfeeding and your baby was gaining weight well on the breast alone. The key to keeping your milk production steady after returning to work is keeping your total number of daily milk removals (breastfeedings plus pumpings) stable during the long term.

Why? The two main dynamics affecting long-term milk production are *degree of breast fullness* and *breast storage capacity*.

Degree of Breast Fullness

This boils down to a very simple concept: drained breasts make milk faster and full breasts make milk slower. Whenever your breasts become full, milk production slows. Full breasts exert pressure within the breasts, which signals your body to slow milk production. The fuller your breasts become, the stronger the signal your body receives to slow milk production.

The opposite is also true. Milk production speeds when your breasts are drained more fully. At an average breastfeeding, baby takes about two-thirds of the milk in the breast and leaves one-third. During the first month of life, to increase your milk production your baby feeds more often and longer, taking a larger percentage of the available milk. This happens very naturally when you're with your baby and feeding on cue.

Another variable related to this concept is your baby's longest sleep stretch, which often increases as your baby gets older. Once you're back at work, if you regularly go longer than eight hours between milk removals, this increases your risk of slowed milk production.

Breast Storage Capacity

The number of milk removals (breastfeedings plus pumpings) needed each day to keep long-term milk production stable (your magic number) varies among mothers because of a physical characteristic known as breast storage capacity. This physical difference explains why feeding patterns can vary so much from one mother and baby to another.

Breast storage capacity simply refers to the most milk available in your breasts when they're at their fullest during the day. Storage capacity is not related to breast size, which is determined mainly by the amount of fatty tissue in the breasts. So smaller-breasted mothers can have a large storage capacity and larger-breasted mothers can have a small capacity.

What effects does this difference in storage capacity have? After baby's first month, while still at home, a mother with a large storage capacity will likely notice a far different breastfeeding pattern compared to the mother with a small storage capacity. Breast storage capacity affects feeding patterns in several ways.

- Whether baby usually takes one breast or both

- Number of feedings needed each day for baby to gain weight well

- Baby's longest sleep stretch

Both large-capacity and small-capacity mothers produce plenty of milk for their babies. Their babies simply feed differently to get the milk they need. A mother with a large storage capacity has more room in her milk-making glands to comfortably hold milk, so it takes more milk to exert the amount of internal pressure that slows milk production. With more milk available in her breasts, her baby may always be satisfied with one breast per feeding. He may gain weight well with fewer feedings per day than most babies. And he may sleep for longer stretches at night without her milk production slowing.

On the other hand, the mother with a small storage capacity will have less milk available at each feeding, so her baby may want both breasts more often, need more feedings each day to get the same amount of milk, and wake often at night to get enough milk. If the baby of the small-capacity mother sleeps for too long, mother's breasts quickly become so full that milk production slows.

If after returning to work your milk production begins to slow, count how many times in each twenty-four-hour day you're removing the milk from your breasts. Chances are your daily number of milk removals has dropped. Maybe your baby has started sleeping longer at night. Maybe you've cut back on breast-feeding while at home. Maybe you're pumping less at work. No matter what the cause, you can reverse this trend by simply increasing your number of daily milk removals. Staying at your magic number should hold your milk production steady. If you increase your number of daily milk removals above your magic number, you can increase your milk production. The following tips describe strategies that have helped many employed mothers.

Breastfeed Often When You're Together

Meeting your long-term breastfeeding goals is easier if you focus on providing most of your baby's milk directly from the breast. Many mothers struggling with milk production pump often enough at work but don't breastfeed often enough when with their babies. Mothers who were breastfeeding eight times per day before they returned to work may be pumping three times at work but only breastfeeding two or three times when with their baby. In other words, during times when they could be breastfeeding, they're not.

What this means in practical terms is that with fewer ses-sions at the breast, baby needs more expressed milk while mother is away, which she has to work harder to provide by pumping. Keep in mind that when you are back at work, your baby will continue to need a fixed amount of milk, on average about 30 ounces (900 mL) per day. The more of those ounces your baby gets directly from the breast while you're together, the less milk you need to express. The opposite is true, too. The less milk your baby gets from the breast, the more milk you'll need to leave for him while you're at work. What's important to a baby is not how much milk he gets at each feeding, but how much milk he gets in each twenty-four-hour day.

How you plan your daily routine can make a world of difference. To maximize your breastfeeding:

- **Breastfeed twice in the morning.** Offer your breast once when you wake up and again right before you leave baby with the caregiver.

- **Breastfeed as soon as you see your baby after work.** If he seems hungry right before you arrive, suggest that the caregiver give as little milk as possible until you get there.

- **Explore the possibility of nursing midday.** See if you can make arrangements to go to your baby for at least one feeding during your workday or have your baby brought to you.

- **Consider other times you can breastfeed.** If your baby starts sleeping longer at night and the overall number of milk removals decreases, think about when you can fit in more breastfeedings at other times.

- **Nurse before bedtime.** If your baby sleeps for longer than eight-hour stretches at night, wake him to breastfeed right before you go to bed or, if you prefer, pump.

Pump More Milk

Several strategies that can help you pump more milk at each session are described in detail in Problem 18. Some involve triggering more milk releases, or *let-downs*, during pumping. These involve varying your pump speed and using your mind and senses to trigger more milk releases (the average number of let-downs during a breastfeeding is five). Milk only flows when you have a milk release. Otherwise the milk stays in your breast.

Making sure your pump suction is the highest that is comfortable (but no higher) can also increase your milk yield, as can *hands-on pumping*, which involves using your hands to massage your breasts and compress them during pumping. Another key strategy is checking your pump fit. If the opening your nipple is pulled into during pumping is too large or small, this can result in less milk pumped. See chapter 6 for illustrations you can use to check your pump fit.

Expect Less Milk After Starting Solids

Solid foods take the place of your milk in your baby's diet. This means that after your baby starts eating solids, his need for milk decreases. It also means that your milk production will likely decrease, even if his total number of feedings does not. Many babies simply take less milk at each feeding (remember: full breasts make milk slower).

If your milk production decreases slowly after solids are started but your baby is satisfied, there is no reason to boost your milk production. Most employed mothers stop pumping sometime between their baby's ninth and twelfth months. After one year, baby can drink other types of milk. You can still breastfeed when you're home but, in most cases, there is no need to keep pumping after that.

If These Strategies Don't Work

There are always exceptions to every rule. If you continue to see a decrease in milk production despite trying all these strategies, know that some mothers simply don't respond to breast pumps in the same way as other mothers. In this case, hand expression may be a better option; the skin-to-skin contact can be more effective for some mothers in triggering milk releases. To see online videos of hand-expression techniques, go to: newborns .stanford.edu/Breastfeeding/HandExpression.html and ammeh jelpen.no/handmelking?id=907 (scroll down for the English version).

Also keep in mind that some breastfeeding is always better than none. Even if you are not able to reach your goal of exclusive breastfeeding, providing your milk for some feedings is still a huge boon to your and your baby's health.

Chapter 3

Nipple Pain

Should breastfeeding be completely pain free or is nipple pain normal? That's important to know, because some women breastfeed in pain for weeks and even months, believing that pain is a normal part of nursing their baby. To be clear on this, the only type of nipple pain you should live with is discomfort during the first minute or two of breastfeeding during your baby's first two weeks of life.

Toe-curling pain when baby latches is not normal. Neither is pain that lasts throughout or between feedings. Consider severe, long-lasting pain or broken skin and color changes on your nipple as problems needing a solution. The good news is that the vast majority of mothers who seek breastfeeding help for nipple pain quickly achieve comfortable breastfeeding. This is

Myth: Nipple pain is a normal part of breastfeeding.

Reality: In the first week or two after birth, most moms have some tenderness during the first minute or so of breastfeeding that quickly subsides when their milk starts flowing, but more-severe nipple pain or pain that persists longer than two weeks is a sign that some adjustment is needed.

true of early nipple pain as well as nipple pain that starts after a period of comfortable breastfeeding and pain related to teething or biting in the older baby.

Problem 8: Your nipples hurt when you breastfeed your newborn or young infant.

Some believe that the mild nipple discomfort considered normal at the very beginning of a feed during the first two weeks is due to greater breast and nipple sensitivity from hormonal changes associated with giving birth. But if your discomfort lasts longer than two weeks, lasts throughout the feeding, or is intense rather than mild, this section is for you.

Some mothers live with painful breastfeeding for months under the assumption that their nipples will "toughen up." However, experienced breastfeeding mothers do not develop nipple calluses, so this idea is simply wrong. What *does* happen over time, though, is that babies develop more head-and-neck control that allows them to latch themselves onto the breast deeper. This means that even without the suggestions in this section, nipple pain and trauma may eventually go away on its own. But why wait when these tips may increase your comfort immediately?

Aim for the Comfort Zone

The most common solution to painful nipples is to get a deeper latch. The deeper your nipple extends into your baby's mouth during feedings, the more comfortable breastfeeding should feel.

To gauge how deep is deep enough, the concept of the *comfort zone* may help. The comfort zone is a real place in your baby's mouth (at the arrow in figure 3-1.) You can find it in your own mouth by running your tongue or your finger along the roof (palate) of your mouth. The section of your palate nearest your front teeth is ridged. Behind these ridges is a smooth area, your hard palate. Closer to your throat, the roof of your mouth becomes soft. The comfort zone is near that area in your baby's mouth, where his palate turns from hard to soft.

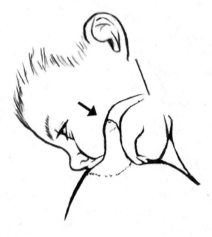

Figure 3-1. For comfortable breastfeeding, your nipple should reach the "comfort zone."

©2012 Peter Mohrbacher, used with permission.

Reaching the comfort zone during breastfeeding protects your nipple from friction and compression, and your baby gets more milk with each suck.

With a shallow latch, your baby's tongue compresses your nipple against his hard palate, causing nipple distortion and pain. You can see nipple distortion when your nipple emerges from your baby's mouth oddly shaped, smashed looking, or pointed, like a new tube of lipstick. If your baby breastfeeds with a shallow latch feeding after feeding, you may get a "compression stripe" on your nipple, which eventually leads to cracks and bleeding. Other types of trauma can occur, too, sometimes looking like a starburst or scabbing on the nipple.

Regular use of bottles and pacifiers during your baby's early weeks can contribute to *superficial nipple sucking*, another term for a shallow latch.

Try to Latch More Deeply

How can you help your baby get a deeper latch? If you breastfeed sitting up or lying on your side, this involves making sure baby's body is pressed against yours (no gaps) and bringing his chin into contact with your breast, either with a light, soft touch or a tapping movement. This contact between breast and chin should trigger a wide-open mouth. Once he opens wide, apply gentle pressure from behind his shoulders as he latches to gently push the breast deeper into his mouth. It may also help him reach the comfort zone if he approaches the breast off-center, so his lower jaw is farther from the nipple than his upper jaw (figure 3-2). That allows the nipple to extend deeper than if you center it when latching.

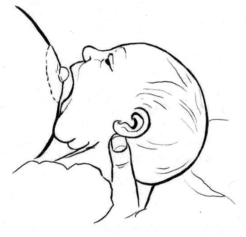

Figure 3-2. For a deeper latch when sitting up, align baby to the breast with his lower jaw as far from the nipple as possible.

©2012 Anna Mohrbacher, used with permission.

An even easier way to get a deeper latch is to use laid-back feeding positions. To do this, lean back far enough so baby is completely supported tummy down on your body but upright enough that you can see him easily without straining your neck (figure 1-1). See "Try Laid-Back Breastfeeding" in chapter 1 for further instructions and illustrations.

Myth: Getting a deep latch can be complicated and frustrating.

Reality: Latching a newborn can feel complicated if you're sitting up or lying on your side, because you have to work to counteract gravity, which pulls your baby down and away from you. Semi-reclined, or laid-back, breastfeeding positions make getting a deep latch easier and more automatic during the newborn period because gravity works in harmony with your baby's inborn feeding behaviors.

73

In fact, reviewing all of the strategies in Problem 1 can help you to achieve a deeper latch.

You'll know you have reached the comfort zone when breastfeeding feels more comfortable than before. If you have nipple trauma, breastfeeding may not yet feel completely comfortable. But any reduction in pain indicates baby has a deeper latch. By getting your nipple into the comfort zone at every breastfeeding, your nipples can heal even while continuing to breastfeed. When there is no more friction or pressure on your nipple, your nipples can heal.

If you are still in pain even after working on getting a deeper latch, check out the next several easy-to-correct causes. If none of these tips helps, it's time to seek skilled breastfeeding help. If a breastfeeding caregiver tells you that your latch looks fine, please get a second (or third) opinion. Your latch may *look* fine, but how it looks is not important. If you are in pain, something needs to be adjusted. Breastfeeding is not supposed to hurt!

Break Suction Before Removing Baby from the Breast

This is one possible cause of nipple pain other than a shallow latch. If you don't break the suction in baby's mouth before removing him from the breast, nipple trauma may result. To remove baby safely and comfortably, slide your little finger into the corner of his mouth between his gums until the suction is broken. Then remove your breast from baby's mouth.

Stop Using Any Breast Pump That Hurts

Just like breastfeeding, breast pumping should always feel comfortable. There are two main reasons a breast pump might hurt you: suction that is too strong or a poor fit. Some of the discount breast pumps generate a suction so powerful that they can damage your nipples. Even when using a high-quality pump, it's possible to set its suction too high. (Always set your suction to the highest setting that's comfortable and no higher.) A "tight fit" can also contribute to pain. If your nipple rubs along the tunnel inside the pump's nipple opening, contact the pump manufacturer and ask if a larger size is available. See also "Make Sure Your Pump Fits" in chapter 6. Don't keep using a pump if it hurts.

Use Comfort Measures

While exploring solutions for your nipple pain, these strategies may help increase your comfort.

- Take pain medication, such as ibuprofen or another analgesic your health care provider recommends.

- Offer your less sore breast first, and switch to the more painful breast after your milk begins to flow. Most mothers find breastfeeding less painful when their milk is flowing.

- Feed more often so that baby is not ravenous when he goes to the breast.

- Try different breastfeeding positions to see if one will hurt less until help arrives.

- Change feeding positions frequently so that one area is not consistently traumatized.

- Use ultrapurified lanolin or hydrogel pads to treat trauma and reduce pain (see "Treat Nipple Trauma").

- Use a nipple shield. These soft silicone shields are worn over your nipple during feedings; your milk flows through the holes in the tip. For some women, the shield provides just enough protection between baby's mouth and mother's skin to make continued breastfeeding tolerable.

- Take a break from breastfeeding and pump to let your nipples heal.

Some mothers find that pumping hurts less than breastfeeding. If your nipples are severely damaged or infected, you may prefer to pump your breasts and feed your baby your milk another way until your nipples heal a bit. But be careful. A poorly designed pump may cause more damage and make things worse, so be sure to use a good-quality, effective pump that fits you well. If you have a newborn, plan to drain your breasts at least eight times each day to prevent painful breast fullness and provide the milk your baby needs.

Treat Nipple Trauma

Nipple trauma is not a normal part of breastfeeding, so don't just ignore it and hope it goes away on its own. As with any broken skin, wash your traumatized nipples with soap and water at least daily in the shower to help prevent infection. But since overzealous cleaning of your breasts or nipples can cause nipple pain, don't overdo it.

Avoid topical creams or ointments that need to be wiped off before breastfeeding. (The better brands of the ultrapurified lanolin, recommended as a trauma treatment, do not need to be removed before nursing.) Also avoid breast pads or bras with plastic liners that can trap moisture.

There are products you can use to ease your pain and speed healing, but your problem will not be completely resolved until you correct its cause. (Although some recommend rubbing expressed milk into the area, this has not been found to help.) In years past, nursing mothers were told to keep their traumatized nipple dry, but all wounds heal faster when kept slightly moist (but not too moist). The following products, which provide a moist-wound-healing environment for your skin, will *not* solve your problem if you continue breastfeeding with a shallow latch, but they can reduce pain and speed healing. How does this work? Keeping broken skin slightly moist keeps your nerve endings in a more normal environment and prevents scabbing, which slows healing. There's no extra benefit to using these products together, so pick one.

Myth: You should never use soap on your nipples.

Reality: If your skin is intact and healthy, there's no reason to wash your nipples with soap, as your breasts secrete an antibacterial fluid. But if you have broken skin, as with any cut or scrape, it's advisable to wash it at least daily with soap and water to help prevent infection.

Lanolin

Ultrapurified lanolin is available at most drug and grocery stores. Check the package. The brands safest for baby do not need to be washed off before the next feeding, so read the packaging. For best results, apply enough lanolin after every feeding to keep your nipples moist until baby breastfeeds again.

If clothing friction bothers you, apply lanolin and wear hard plastic breast shells, which can be found in most large baby stores (see Resources for product links), in your bra between feedings to protect your nipples. When using breast shells, be sure your bra cup is large enough to hold them in place without leaving red rings on your breasts when removed.

Hydrogel Pads

Hydrogel pads are available at most baby and drug stores. Some mothers find that they reduce nipple pain more than ultrapurified lanolin. Brand names include Soothies, Ameda ComfortGel, and Medela Tender Care. Wear these soothing gel pads in your bra between feedings. For even greater comfort, chill them in the refrigerator before putting them on. They can be reused until they turn cloudy, when they should be discarded. Follow the care instructions that come with your hydrogels, as they vary from brand to brand. Some brands last much longer than others so check the wear time when choosing.

If These Strategies Don't Work

Other possible reasons for nipple pain and trauma are less common. If the previous suggestions don't help, consider the following.

Unusual Anatomy in You or Your Baby

Although an uncommon cause of nipple pain, consider unusual anatomy in your or your baby.

Inverted Nipples

An inverted nipple looks like it's inside out, even when stimulated. Think of it as an *innie* rather than an *outie*. Most babies can breastfeed just fine from inverted nipples, but if your nipples have not spent much time pulled out, the first time this skin is stimulated during nursing, it may cause discomfort. The skin that is not usually exposed may even look red or raw after breastfeeding. If your pain is mild, it will likely decrease over time. If severe, try breast pumping; if pumping feels more comfortable, some time spent pumping, either part-time or exclusively, may make your transition to breastfeeding easier. To reach full milk production while pumping exclusively, which is about 25 to 30 ounces (750 to 900 mL) per day, pump at least eight times each day at first until you get there, ideally within the first two weeks after birth.

Large Nipples/Small Mouth

If there is a size mismatch between your nipples and your baby's mouth, take heart. It is only temporary. At first it may be difficult or impossible for your small-mouthed baby to latch on deeply to your very large nipples, but this challenge is quickly outgrown, usually within a few weeks. Baby's mouth will soon become large enough to latch deeply. In the meantime, you can establish full milk production with an effective breast pump (see "Inverted Nipples") and feed your baby your milk.

Tongue-Tie

This term refers to a short *frenulum*, the stringy membrane that connects your baby's tongue to the floor of his mouth. If baby's frenulum is short near the tip of his tongue, it may prevent him from extending his tongue over his lower gum during feedings. (Have a helper check for this while you're breastfeeding.) Other types of tongue-tie restrict the movement of the back or middle of baby's tongue, causing pain for you and/or making the tongue movements needed for effective breastfeeding impossible. Indicators of tongue-tie may include one or more of the following:

- Nipple pain or trauma, despite a deep latch

- Clicking sounds and/or difficulty staying on the breast

- Slow weight gain

If you suspect your baby is tongue-tied, take a look at his tongue when his mouth is open. As he tries to stick it out, its tip may indent in the middle, forming a heart shape. Or he may be unable to raise either the back or the front of his tongue to the roof of his mouth.

The most effective treatment for tongue-tie is to release baby's frenulum by clipping it. That sounds worse than it is, because there are few nerves and blood vessels in the frenulum, and the procedure is usually done quickly in a doctor's office with little or no need for anesthesia. After this procedure, your baby should be able to nurse immediately. You will likely notice an amazing decrease in pain while your baby is at breast. Health professionals who may perform this procedure include oral surgeons, dentists, pediatricians, family-practice doctors, and ear, nose, and throat specialists. Ask the breastfeeding specialists in your community who performs this procedure in your area. These health care professionals should be able to determine the need for it as well as do it. If a tongue-tied baby is able to breastfeed effectively and comfortably, there is no need for this procedure to be performed.

Bacterial and Yeast Infections

Where there's broken skin, infections can occur. Nipple trauma puts you at greater risk for developing a bacterial or yeast infection, as well as *mastitis* (see Problem 13), an inflamed or infected area inside your breast.

How do you know if you have an infection on your nipple? Breastfeeding will suddenly become much more painful and your healing will slow or even stop. This is when you should consider infection as a possibility. Both bacterial and yeast infections can cause severe pain. In some women, the pain is so intense they turn to pumping to avoid putting baby to breast.

Bacterial Infections of the Nipple

In addition to the infection symptoms described above, if your infection is bacterial, you may also see pus or yellow scabbing on your nipple. Most women whose nipple pain continues for weeks have a staph infection of the nipple. The most effective treatment for this is a course of oral antibiotics, nearly all of which are compatible with continued breastfeeding. Oral cloxacillin or erythromycin (for those allergic to penicillin) taken in 500-mg doses every six hours for ten days resolves nipple bacterial infection in nearly 80 percent of women, and this treatment is compatible with breastfeeding. If you'd like to share this information with your health care provider, refer him or her to the V. Livingstone study cited in the Resources section. In some unusual cases, long-term antibiotic treatment may be necessary. If the ten-day course of antibiotics isn't enough to resolve your nipple pain, refer your health care provider to A. Eglash's article in the *Journal of Human Lactation*, which is also cited in the Resources section, for guidance on alternative treatments.

Yeast Infections of the Nipple

Another type of nipple infection is caused by an overgrowth of the yeast *Candida albicans*, which can lead to severe nipple pain often described as "burning" or "shooting." The skin around your nipple may be red, scaly, or flaky, or it may be smooth and shiny. Your nipples may or may not be itchy. The pain may be worse after feeding or at night.

If your baby also has a yeast infection, it may appear as white patches inside his mouth (thrush) or as diaper rash. *Candida albicans* can cause nipple pain even if no thrush is seen in baby's mouth.

If you have a yeast infection of the nipple, both you and your baby need to be treated. See "Get Checked for a Yeast Infection" later in this chapter for treatment options.

Other Skin Problems

Contact dermatitis, impetigo, eczema, and psoriasis can also cause nipple pain. If you're not sure what type of skin problem you have, see a dermatologist for diagnosis and treatment. Nearly all treatments are compatible with continued breastfeeding.

Overabundant Milk Production

How can making too much milk cause nipple pain? When milk flow is overwhelming, baby may compress or crimp the nipple to slow it down and make it more manageable. You can rule this in or out by considering your baby's weight gain. Average weight gain during baby's first three to four months is about 2 pounds per month. Babies of mothers with overabundant milk production typically gain double that or more.

What can you do if that's the problem? Try laid-back breastfeeding positions (figure 1-1), as gravity may help baby better control milk flow without the need to compress the nipple. If that doesn't help, see the strategies for dealing with Problem 6.

Problem 9: Your nipples hurt between feedings.

The two most common causes of nipple pain between feedings are pain from nipple trauma and restricted blood flow to the nipple from *vasospasm* or *Raynaud's phenomenon*.

Treat Nipple Trauma

If you have nipple trauma and pain during breastfeeding, you may also experience pain between feedings. If so, the first step is to correct the cause of the pain, which is most commonly a shallow latch. See "Get a Deeper Latch" earlier in this chapter for strategies.

After correcting the cause of your nipple damage, consider using either lanolin (see "Lanolin" earlier in this chapter) or hydrogel pads (see "Hydrogel Pads" earlier in this chapter). Both products keep your wound slightly moist, which reduces pain and speeds healing by preventing scabbing.

Check Your Nipples After Nursing for Color Changes

There are two conditions that restrict blood flow to the nipple and can cause pain between feedings: vasospasm and Raynaud's phenomenon. The specific color changes you may see after breastfeedings, in conjunction with your health history, can help you and your health care provider determine which condition is causing your pain.

Vasospasm is characterized by nipples turning white after a feeding, along with pain. A deeper latch is one remedy. Raynaud's phenomenon is characterized by nipples turning white, blue, and/or red, along with shooting breast pain between feedings. To read more about these conditions and their treatment suggestions, see "Check for Changes in Nipple Color" in chapter 4.

If These Strategies Don't Work

Another possible cause of nipple pain between feedings is called *referred pain*. This occurs when a painful injury or condition shares the same nerve pathways as your nipple, causing you to perceive pain elsewhere in your body as nipple pain. *Mastitis*, which may cause breast pain, can cause referred nipple pain (see Problem 13). Other conditions include a pulled muscle in your back, neck, or shoulders, or fibromyalgia. Treatment for the underlying condition or the use of pain medications can relieve referred pain.

Keep in mind that continuing pain is not normal. Don't settle for a painful experience. If the strategies in this chapter have not solved your problem, it's time to get the skilled help and support your deserve.

Problem 10: Your nipples start to hurt after a period of comfortable breastfeeding.

As your baby gets older and becomes more coordinated, he needs less help to achieve a deep latch. But an active baby may sometimes stretch your nipple, which can affect your comfort. If baby's movements at the breast cause nipple pain, it's okay to set limits on how he breastfeeds.

Break the Suction If Baby Becomes Distracted

As babies grow and become more aware of their surroundings, even while feeding they may turn their heads to look at distractions without first releasing the breast. Ouch! Regular nipple stretching can lead to soreness and damage. If so, be ready to break the suction. Over time, consistent removal from the breast discourages this behavior.

Tip: To remove baby safely and comfortably from the breast, slide your finger into the corner of his mouth between his gums until the suction is broken and he releases your nipple. Then put him back on again, positioning him to latch as deeply as possible.

Go Back to Basics for a Deeper Latch

If your baby is learning to crawl or walk, he may breastfeed in all sorts of unusual positions, some of which may verge on the acrobatic. When he stretches and moves during breastfeeding, he may pull on your nipple and cause pain. Keep in mind that breastfeeding is a two-way street. It must be good for both of you. There's nothing wrong with letting your baby know that he can breastfeed only in ways that are comfortable for you.

This might involve going back to basics and helping your baby get a nice deep latch when he takes the breast. This might also involve restricting breastfeeding to positions in which baby stays in one spot and doesn't pull on your breast. One way to do this is to breastfeed in a darkened room where there are no distractions. If baby stretches your nipple uncomfortably, break the suction with your finger to teach him that's not okay.

Get Checked for a Yeast Infection

One common cause of nipple pain after a period of comfortable breastfeeding is a yeast infection known as *thrush* or *candidiasis*. It is an overgrowth of the yeast *Candida albicans*, which thrives in moist, dark places, such as on the nipples, in the vagina, in the mouth, and in the baby's diaper area. It normally lives in our bodies in balance with other organisms, but illness, pregnancy, antibiotic use, or other factors that throw the body out of balance can cause an unhealthy overgrowth. A yeast infection may also be passed to you from your baby.

Your Symptoms

Shooting pains in your breasts between feedings are unlikely to be caused by a yeast infection if that is your only symptom. With breast pain alone, a bacterial infection is three times more likely. But a yeast infection is a possible cause if you have these symptoms together:

- Shiny skin on and around your nipple along with breast pain

- Flaky skin on and around your nipple along with breast pain

- Nipples that are itchy along with breast pain

Your Baby's Symptoms

Your baby may not have symptoms, but if he does, they might include:

- White patches on the baby's gums, cheeks, palate, tonsils, and/or tongue (if wiped off, they may look red or bleed)

- Diaper rash (may be simply red or red with raised dots)

Most breastfed babies have a white, milky coating on their tongue. This is not a sign of a yeast infection unless white patches spread to your baby's cheeks and gums. Some babies can have a yeast rash on their bottom but not in their mouth.

Treatments

If a yeast infection is diagnosed by a health care provider, it's important for both you and your baby to be treated or you are likely to reinfect each other. You may also need to treat any other family members (including your partner) if they have symptoms of yeast overgrowth.

Treatment options for you include nystatin cream or ointment (which is much less effective at eradicating yeast than other treatments due to its common and long-term use); gentian violet (a 0.5% or 1% solution applied to your nipple area with a cotton swab once per day for four to seven days); over-the-counter antifungal creams such as clotrimazole (sold as Mycelex, Lotrimin, Lotrimin AF cream or lotion [1%]), miconazole (sold as Micatin, Monistat-Derm cream or lotion [2%]), and ketoconazole (sold as Nizoral); and nystatin with triamcinolone (a corticosteroid). It is not necessary to wipe these treatments off before breastfeeding.

Treatment options for your baby include nystatin suspension (less effective than other treatments) swabbed in baby's mouth four to eight times per day, gentian violet (a 0.5% or 1.0% solution either swabbed in baby's mouth or applied to your nipple area followed by immediate breastfeeding once or twice a day for four to seven days), oral clotrimazole, and oral fluconazole. Antifungal diaper ointments may be recommended for a diaper rash.

If you have a mild case, you may begin to feel relief after one to two days of treatment. With more severe cases, it can take three to five days. If you take oral fluconazole, it may take a week or longer for the pain to disappear, because rather than killing the yeast, it prevents it from reproducing. To prevent recurrence, be sure to do the full course of treatment.

Check Your Nipples for a Blister or a White Spot

Both a nipple blister and a white spot (also known as a *bleb*) can be very painful. Their causes are different but their treatments are similar.

Nipple Blister

Caused by friction and strong suction, a blister may form on the face of the nipple if baby is breastfeeding shallowly and putting pressure on its tip. Helping baby latch more deeply may be all that's needed to reduce the pain and prevent the blister from recurring.

If the blister is very painful, opening it may relieve the pain. To open a blister, apply warm, wet compresses before breastfeeding. The moisture will soften the blister and the heat will thin the skin, which may cause the blister to open. If not, see your health care provider about opening it.

To prevent infection in an opened blister, wash the opened blister at least once a day with soap and water (such as while in the shower). You may also use an over-the-counter antibiotic ointment like Polysporin after breastfeeding. As long as the topical ointment is applied sparingly, it does not need to be rinsed off before the next breastfeeding.

White Spot (Bleb)

If the white spot on your nipple is not painful, you don't have to do anything about it. But if it hurts, treating it can make breastfeeding more comfortable. Possible causes of a nipple bleb include a plugged milk pore from thickened milk in the breast or skin blocking the milk duct.

If the bleb hurts, before breastfeeding apply wet heat by either soaking your nipple in water by lying on your side in a warm tub or leaning over a basin, or by applying moist, warm compresses. The idea is to thin the skin so that the baby can more easily draw out the plug of thickened milk during breastfeeding. If the bleb is not relieved with wet heat and breastfeeding:

- Wear a cotton ball soaked with olive oil placed over the spot in your bra between feedings to soften the skin.

- Once the skin is softened, try to peel away any thickened skin over the bleb and then try to manually express the plug.

If these strategies don't bring relief, ask your health care provider to open the bleb. You should see immediate milk flow. If the bleb is dry and the milk doesn't flow, continue trying the suggestions above.

If you have a problem with recurring blebs, try eliminating saturated fats from your diet and take lecithin supplements (1 tablespoon three times per day or one or two 1,200-mg capsules three or four times per day).

Some mothers report a white spot on their nipple after the baby has bitten them, which is caused by an accumulation of saliva and milk moisture under skin edges. In this case, treat it like any bite wound by washing gently with soap and water.

If These Strategies Don't Work

The following are other possible causes of sudden-onset nipple pain.

- **Trauma caused by a breast pump.** A wide variety of breast pumps are on the market. Yours may have a poor fit or a too-high suction setting, both of which can cause skin trauma and pain. See "Make Sure Your Pump Fits" in chapter 6 for solutions.

- **Products that cause nipple irritation.** Cleaning your breasts or nipples with alcohol or washing with soap too frequently can cause nipple irritation. Read "Avoid Products that Irritate Your Nipples" earlier in this chapter for additional items known to cause nipple pain and to learn about what alternatives exist.

- **Pregnancy.** The hormonal changes of pregnancy can cause nipple pain. In fact, nearly three-quarters of pregnant women report nipple tenderness and discomfort during pregnancy, and this pain may be one of the first symptoms. It's not possible to change your hormones, but helping baby get a deep latch has helped many pregnant women achieve more comfortable breastfeeding.

- **Teething.** Is your baby teething? If so, see the next section.

Problem 11: Your baby is teething and has bitten you.

Many mothers are warned to wean before baby's first tooth appears. However, many babies never bite, and those who bite once usually never bite again. Keep in mind that while baby is actively nursing, she can't bite, because her tongue covers her lower gum. It may also help to know that nipple pain caused by a teething baby will pass as her teeth erupt. Some teething babies bear down, chew on the nipple (pressure feels good on sore, swollen gums), or bite. The following strategies may help you prevent or ease the pain from both teething and biting.

Myth: You should wean before your baby gets teeth.

Reality: Many babies never bite, and nearly all of those who do can be taught not to. Most babies cut their first teeth between eight and twelve months (and some much earlier—some are born with teeth!). Since breastfeeding (with solid foods added at six months) is recommended for a minimum of one year, don't wean simply because you fear a tooth is coming in.

Use Cold to Numb Baby's Gums Before Breastfeeding

If baby's gums are numb, she is less likely to bear down or chew on you to ease her discomfort. To numb her gums, before offering the breast give baby something cold to chew on, such as:

- A cold, wet washcloth

- A refrigerated teething toy

- A frozen food such as a bagel or frozen peas, if baby has started solids

Consult with your baby's health care provider before using an over-the-counter teething preparation to numb her gums. These products may also numb baby's tongue (and your breast!), making breastfeeding difficult.

Learn How to Discourage Biting

Most mothers' first reaction to the baby bearing down on or biting the nipple is to startle and pull baby off the breast. After this reaction, most babies never bite again. But if a baby does bite again, try to stay calm. Pulling baby off the breast with her teeth clamped down can cause more damage than the bite itself.

The following strategies may help discourage a persistent biter.

- **Stop the feeding.** Remove the temptation for baby to make you jump.

- **Offer something else to bite on.** A teething ring, toy, or anything acceptable to bite can suffice.

- **Set baby quickly on the floor.** This gives the message that biting brings negative consequences. After a few seconds of distress, comfort baby.

- **Keep a finger near baby's mouth ready to break the suction.** Some distractible babies try to turn and look with the nipple still in their mouth. If you respond consistently by breaking the suction, baby will learn quickly that turning away means losing the nipple.

- **Make sure baby latches deeply.** Being well onto the breast triggers active suckling and lessens the odds of biting.

Try to Reduce Your Discomfort

While experimenting with strategies to discourage bearing down or biting, try the following to reduce your pain.

- **Take pain medication** such as ibuprofen (which also reduces inflammation) or another analgesic that your health care provider recommends.

- **Offer your less sore breast first**, and then switch to the other after your milk is flowing. Most mothers find breastfeeding less painful after their milk lets down.

- **Try varying feeding positions** so that one area is not consistently traumatized.

- **Use ultrapurified lanolin or hydrogel pads** to reduce pain.

- **Take a break from breastfeeding and pumping** to let your nipples heal.

If your nipples are severely damaged, you may prefer to pump your breasts and feed your baby by cup or bottle until your nipples heal a bit. Some mothers find that pumping hurts less than breastfeeding. Just remember to drain your breasts at least six times a day to prevent painful breast fullness and provide milk for your baby.

If These Strategies Don't Work

If your baby has been biting persistently, try the following strategies:

- **Give baby your complete attention during breastfeeding.** Eye contact, stroking, and talking decrease the odds that baby will bite to get your attention.

- **Learn to recognize the end of a feeding.** Most biting occurs when baby loses interest in breastfeeding. You may notice, for example, that tension develops in baby's jaw before she bites down. When you see this sign, you can break the suction and take her off before she bites.

- **Don't pressure a disinterested baby to breastfeed.** If baby pushes you away, offer the breast again later.

- **Remove a sleeping baby who's no longer actively suckling.** To do this, gently insert your finger between baby's gums to release the nipple. If baby bites, she'll bite the finger instead of your breast.

- **Keep your milk production abundant.** Some babies bite when they are frustrated by too little milk.

- **Note behaviors that lead to biting.** Some babies bite when teased or when you raise your voice to older siblings. Notice what happens before baby bites. Knowing the trigger may help you prevent future biting.

- **Keep breastfeeding relaxed and positive.** Some babies bite when mother is tense. If you feel frazzled, try deep breathing, listening to relaxing music, or breastfeeding while lying down or in a darkened room.

- **Give praise when baby doesn't bite.** Say "thank you" and "good baby" when she is gentle at the breast. Smiles, hugs, and kisses are loving ways to help teach baby to breastfeed comfortably.

Baby needs to learn what to do with new teeth while breastfeeding. Babies don't understand that biting causes pain. They don't bite because of "meanness." Breastfeeding babies learn to associate their mother with feelings of security and comfort, as well as relief from hunger. When these positive associations are suddenly disrupted by baby's biting, baby should learn quickly not to do it again.

Chapter 4

Breast Pain

If breast pain is your challenge, this chapter is for you. Breast pain during the first week or so after birth is usually caused by *engorgement*, which most moms can quickly relieve with prompt treatment. Breast pain at other times is most often due to *mastitis*, also known as a plugged duct or breast infection, which one in five breastfeeding mothers experiences at some point. Other types of infections and circulatory problems can also cause breast pain. And all of these challenges can be overcome. Read on for tips to help you achieve comfortable breastfeeding.

Problem 12: Engorgement—a few days after giving birth, your breasts are swollen and painful.

Early engorgement occurs when several bodily fluids—blood, lymph, and milk—converge in the postpartum breast. IV fluids given during labor can also contribute to breast (and ankle) swelling. By using the treatments below, breast engorgement should subside within a day or two.

Take an Anti-Inflammatory Medication

An over-the-counter anti-inflammatory, such as ibuprofen, is considered the most effective treatment for engorgement and is compatible with breastfeeding. Anti-inflammatories also act as pain relievers to reduce your discomfort. Ask your health care provider to recommend one.

Myth: You shouldn't take any medications while breastfeeding.

Reality: The vast majority of over-the-counter and prescribed medications are considered *compatible with breastfeeding*. According to the experts, this means that the health risks of feeding your baby formula are considered greater than continuing to breastfeed baby with a miniscule amount of that drug in your milk. Often the only protection your baby receives from your health problem is in your milk. This protection comes from the antibodies that your body adds to your milk whenever you are exposed to an illness of any kind, as well as other milk components that keep your baby healthy.

Remove Your Milk Well and Often

Many mothers worry that more frequent breastfeeding or pumping will worsen breast engorgement by increasing their milk production. But because there is more to engorgement than milk, the opposite is true. Removing the milk from your breasts allows blood and lymph to drain more easily, relieving breast congestion faster.

Breastfeed Eight to Twelve Times Each Day

Try to keep your breasts well drained of milk by breastfeeding at least every hour and a half to two hours during the day and at least every two to three hours at night until your engorgement is gone. Make sure your baby has a deep latch so that he gets more milk more quickly. If your baby's sucking slows down during breastfeeding, try compressing your breast to speed milk flow.

Avoid Bottles and Pacifiers

If your baby is breastfeeding well, to relieve your engorgement faster keep him at the breast for all feeding opportunities. A pacifier delays feedings, which will only make engorgement worse.

If your baby is not breastfeeding well, use the other chapters in this book to help determine a cause—and don't give up! If you need to pump to relieve engorgement and feed your baby another way until latching is easier, then do so—there's no reason to feel bad about it. You can put baby back on the breast as soon as your problem is resolved.

Express Milk

If your baby is not breastfeeding yet, plan to pump as often as he would be breastfeeding, at least every hour and a half to two hours during the day and at least every two to three hours at night, until your engorgement has subsided.

If your baby is not breastfeeding well enough to relieve your breast fullness, and you have an effective breast pump, try just once to drain the milk from both breasts as fully as possible. If needed, do it more than once. This may help you turn the corner.

If your engorgement comes and goes or is mild or moderate, another strategy is to *pump to comfort*, which means pumping just long enough to feel more comfortable rather than trying to drain your breasts completely. Pump only when you feel full and baby does not relieve this fullness. At some feedings your baby may be full after one breast, leaving your unused breast feeling hard or swollen. In this case, pump the unused side.

Try Reverse-Pressure Softening

Engorgement can sometimes cause the dark circle around your nipple (areola) to feel firm rather than soft. This can lead to a shallow latch, which can mean nipple pain for you and less milk for your baby. *Reverse-pressure softening* (RPS) is an easy way to make this area very soft right before feedings so that your baby can latch deeply and comfortably. See "Use Reverse-Pressure Softening If Your Breasts Feel Firm" in chapter 1 for details on how to perform this technique, along with handy illustrations.

Apply Cold or Warmth to Your Breasts

Use whichever feels best, or alternate coolness and heat at different times. A warm shower or warm compresses right before breastfeeding may help the milk flow, but don't overdo it: too much warmth can increase inflammation. Cold reduces inflammation, so between feedings wrap a towel around crushed ice, a reusable soft ice pack, or a bag of frozen peas or corn and hold it to the breast for fifteen to twenty minutes at a time.

Wear a Supportive Bra

Again, let your comfort be your guide. When their breasts are in this large and swollen state, many mothers feel more comfortable when their breasts are well supported. Otherwise the weight of their breasts may cause muscle strain. Try wearing a sports bra or any bra that provides good support. If it feels good, you can even wear one at night. Avoid bras that are too tight, since consistent compression on the breast can cause a type of mastitis known as *plugged ducts*, a painful, hardened area in your breast.

If You Have a Fever, Contact Your Health Care Provider

If your temperature is above 100.6°F (38.4°C) and/or you are having any flu-like symptoms, along with being engorged, call your health care provider. You may have developed *mastitis* (see Problem 13), which may need to be treated.

If These Strategies Don't Work

A home remedy for engorgement that some mothers swear by is cabbage leaves. Yes, you heard that right! Rinse refrigerated or room-temperature green cabbage leaves, crush the large vein with your hands or with a rolling pin, and cut a hole for your nipple. Apply these leaves directly to your breasts and wear them inside your bra. After two to four hours, remove them and apply fresh leaves. If they work, you should notice improvement within a day.

If you are still very engorged, keep in mind that there are other breast conditions, such as mastitis, that may be mistaken for engorgement, so if your symptoms don't improve with these treatments, see your health care provider to rule them out.

Problem 13: Mastitis—your breast is tender or painful, you feel a lump, and/or you're running a fever.

Mastitis refers to an inflamed area in the breast with or without a fever. A mild form of mastitis—a tender spot or lump in your breast with no fever—is sometimes called a *plugged* or *clogged duct*. Mastitis can be mild or severe, from the breast lump that goes away with one good breastfeeding to a hard, very painful breast with a high fever that requires medical treatment.

Myth: If you develop mastitis, you should stop breastfeeding.

Reality: Most cases of mastitis can be quickly resolved with either home treatment or antibiotics, so it is not necessary to wean. In fact, weaning during mastitis is not recommended because it puts you at risk for more serious complications, such as a *breast abscess*. This is a walled-off area of pus within the breast that usually requires surgical drainage and a stay in the hospital, making it well worth avoiding! For this reason, if you want to wean, it's better to do so after the mastitis has completely cleared.

If you have mastitis, the following strategies can help you feel better soon. Basic treatments are the same (with the exception of antibiotics) whether or not your mastitis involves infection.

Take an Anti-Inflammatory Medication

An anti-inflammatory, such as ibuprofen, will help reduce your pain and inflammation. Plus it's compatible with breastfeeding. Ask your health care provider to recommend one.

Remove Your Milk Well and Often

Despite discomfort, which can sometimes be intense during mastitis, continued, frequent breastfeeding is recommended. Allowing your breasts to stay full of milk can cause a case of mastitis to worsen. And milk from a breast with mastitis is perfectly safe for your baby to drink.

To ease your discomfort, try different breastfeeding positions, and for now stick with the one that feels most comfortable. Make sure your baby has a deep latch, as that will help the milk drain better. It may help your mastitis to clear faster if you breastfeed with her nose or chin pointing toward the sore area.

Try to breastfeed at least every two hours during the day and every three hours at night, starting with the sore breast. Breast inflammation causes milk flow to slow from that area. Most mothers with mastitis notice reduced milk production in their affected breast. (Because the breasts make more milk than baby needs, this shouldn't cause problems for baby.)

If your baby refuses to nurse on your affected breast, you will need to pump often on that side until the mastitis clears.

Frequent breastfeeding or pumping will help clear the mastitis more quickly and help boost your milk production back to where it was before your mastitis developed. When pumping, some mothers report seeing the "plug" in their milk in the form of thickened milk or crystals. Again, this is safe to feed the baby.

Apply Warm Compresses and Use Gentle Breast Massage

At least three times each day, apply warm compresses (wet or dry) to the tender area or soak your affected breast in warm water by lying on your side in a tub or by leaning over a basin. Breastfeed or pump right after applying heat to help loosen the plug.

Massage the area with your palm and fingers in a circular motion. You can also use your fingertips to knead your breast, moving from your armpit toward your nipple.

Tip: Avoid tight or restrictive clothing while treating mastitis. If you can comfortably go without a bra, plan to do so for a couple of days whenever possible.

Rest

If you become fatigued and stressed, your body's resistance to infection will decrease. Mastitis may be your body's way of telling you that you are doing too much. Rest as much as you can to allow your body's natural defenses to fight infection. If you find yourself battling recurring mastitis, give yourself some extra downtime while you try to determine what's causing it.

Consider Possible Causes

To avoid getting mastitis again, try to determine the reason you developed it in the first place. The most common causes of mastitis are:

- Broken skin on the nipple, where bacteria can enter the breast

- A too-tight bra or anything that puts consistent pressure on or compresses your breast (sleeping on your stomach, a baby carrier, a strap from a purse or diaper bag)

- Breast(s) staying overly full for too long

Prolonged breast fullness can happen with irregular feeding patterns, a sudden change in feeding frequency (baby begins sleeping through the night), starting supplements by bottle, and pacifier overuse. Too-full breasts can also happen when you're really busy and go longer than usual between feedings (such as during holidays and family gatherings). If any of these situations sound possible, be mindful of them in the future to avoid a recurrence of mastitis.

If These Strategies Don't Work

Most mothers using the home treatments for mastitis in this section can clear it on their own. If your symptoms don't improve within two days, see your health care provider. You may need a different antibiotic or you may have another breast condition that was mistaken for mastitis, such as *cellulitis, galactoceles,* or *cysts.* Most breast conditions are not serious, but it is important to rule out the grave possibilities as well. Call your health care provider when:

- Your temperature spikes above 101°F (38.4°C)
- You feel achy or have other flu-like symptoms
- You see pus in a cracked nipple or red streaks on your breast
- Your milk contains pus or blood
- Any of these symptoms appear suddenly and severely

If you report these symptoms, your health care provider may prescribe an antibiotic. The antibiotics prescribed for mastitis should be compatible with breastfeeding. (If not, ask for some that are.) It is important to take the full course to avoid a recurrence.

Problem 14: You have shooting pains in your breasts between feedings.

Shooting breast pains between feedings have several common causes. To start, look carefully at your nipple for either a change in color or for evidence of trauma. If you have either symptom, read on to figure out what you can do.

Check for Changes in Nipple Color

If your nipples turn white (blanch) when your breast pain starts, this pain may be due to restricted blood flow to your nipples. This can be caused by a temporary condition known as *vasospasm*, or you may have *Raynaud's phenomenon*.

Vasospasm is caused by a constriction of blood vessels, which typically is a result of your baby compressing your nipple against his hard palate due to a shallow latch. Pain from vasospasm continues until blood returns to the nipple. The remedies that follow, along with a deeper latch (see "Get a Deeper Latch" in chapter 2), can help.

Raynaud's phenomenon is a circulatory problem that causes the arteries leading to fingers, toes, and nipples (and sometimes ears, cheeks, and the tip of your nose) to constrict in response to its triggers. These triggers include exposure to cold, compression, caffeine, and some prescribed and over-the-counter medications. Raynaud's phenomenon is more common among women than men and also more common in those with autoimmune disorders, although it can occur alone. Those with Raynaud's phenomenon often have a history of color changes and pain in their fingers or toes after exposure to these triggers. When the nipples are affected, after breastfeeding they may turn white or any combination of white, blue, and red. The blood flowing back to the nipple can cause a burning sensation, intense throbbing, or shooting pain.

Check your nipples for color changes when the pain begins. If you see no change in color, then vasospasm or Raynaud's phenomenon is probably not the cause. If you do see color changes, the following treatments may help.

Apply Warmth to Your Nipples After Breastfeeding

Warmth can prevent or relieve breast pain by quickly increasing blood flow to the nipple. As soon as baby comes off the breast, apply warm compresses, a heating pad, or air from a hair dryer set on warm; take a warm shower; or immerse your breasts in warm water. Dressing warmly and avoiding nipple exposure to air may also help. Some moms find it helps to wear thick nursing pads made from natural fibers to keep their nipples warm.

Tip: You can quickly increase blood flow to the nipple by using gentle nipple massage right after baby releases the breast. This should also help ease any pain.

Avoid Exposure to Cold and Other Triggers

For some mothers, staying warm and avoiding cold air is enough to prevent breast pain after feedings. This may include breastfeeding with a blanket wrapped around you. Caffeine, alcohol, nicotine, and emotional stress can cause constriction of the blood vessels, as can some drugs, such as beta-blockers, oral contraceptives, and pseudoephedrine. Avoiding these triggers may also prevent or reduce breast pain.

Another color-change trigger is compression of the nipples from a shallow latch. With a shallow latch, your baby's tongue presses your nipple against his hard palate, causing nipple distortion and reducing blood flow to the nipple. You can see nipple distortion when your nipple emerges from baby's mouth oddly shaped, smashed, or pointed. Getting a deeper latch will reduce pain in women with Raynaud's phenomenon and may even help prevent vasospasm. To achieve a deeper latch, first you will need to get yourself in a semi-reclined feeding posture (see "Try Laid-Back Breastfeeding" in chapter 1 for details and illustrations). Then you will need to help baby get into position. The section "Aim for the Comfort Zone" in chapter 3 provides directions and advice for achieving the deepest latch possible.

You'll know that you have a successful deep latch when your breast pain decreases or disappears. If your pain does not change, try the other tips in this section.

Take Over-the-Counter Pain Medication

An over-the-counter pain reliever, such as ibuprofen, should help reduce the pain and is compatible with breastfeeding. Some mothers find that taking over-the-counter analgesics regularly for a while keeps them comfortable and prevents pain. Ask your health care provider to recommend one.

Ask About Prescribed Treatments

If you have Raynaud's phenomenon, ask your health care provider about one of the most effective treatments, nifedipine, a prescribed calcium channel blocker that increases blood flow. The recommended dose of 30 to 60 mg per day of sustained-release formulation is compatible with breastfeeding. A two-week course may be long enough to relieve the pain for most mothers without recurrence, but some may need to take it longer.

Check for Nipple Trauma

If you have nipple trauma that has not yet healed or you had nipple trauma in the past, this may be the underlying cause of your breast pain. Mothers with nipple damage may develop complications that cause breast pain, such as referred pain, bacterial or yeast infections, or a combination of the three. Infection can develop anywhere there is broken skin. Most nipple infections are bacterial, but some moms develop yeast infections on their nipples, and both can cause breast pain.

Rule out Referred Pain

The term *referred pain* describes pain from an injury that travels along the body's nerve pathways and is felt in another location. In this case, pain from nipple trauma may be felt as breast pain. Although perceived as breast pain, its cause is nipple damage. You will know this is the cause of your breast pain if the ache stops after your nipple heals. (See "Treat Nipple Trauma" in chapter 3 for healing tips.)

Rule Out a Bacterial Infection

Bacterial and fungal infections have some symptoms in common, but a bacterial infection is much more likely. If your traumatized nipples are healing unusually slowly, healing has stopped, or your nipple or breast pain intensifies despite efforts to correct its cause, the most likely reason is a nipple bacterial infection. In addition to slowed healing and increasing pain, you may see pus or a yellow scab on your nipple.

Antibiotic ointments can help *prevent* bacterial infection where there is broken skin, but topical treatments are not very effective in treating infection after it has developed. Only about one-third of nipple bacterial infections improve when treated with ointments.

The most effective treatment for a nipple bacterial infection is oral antibiotics, which also prevent *mastitis* (a.k.a. plugged ducts and breast infections), another complication of nipple damage. Oral cloxacillin or erythromycin (for those allergic to penicillin) taken in 500-mg doses every six hours for ten days resolves nipple bacterial infection in nearly 80 percent of women, and this treatment is compatible with breastfeeding. Check the Resources section for a study by V. Livingstone on this that you can share with your health care provider. In some unusual cases, long-term antibiotic treatment may be necessary. If the ten-day course of antibiotics isn't enough to resolve your breast pain, refer your health care provider to A. Eglash's article in the *Journal of Human Lactation*, which is also cited in the Resources section, for guidance on alternative treatments.

Rule Out a Yeast Infection

A yeast infection, also known as *thrush* or *candidiasis*, is an overgrowth of a yeast that normally lives in our bodies in balance with other organisms. It typically appears after antibiotic use, which kills the good bacteria in our bodies along with the bad, sending our systems out of balance.

The breast pain associated with a yeast infection may be burning or shooting and is usually intense. The pain may be worse after feedings or at night. Your nipples may or may not be itchy. The skin on your nipple and the surrounding skin may look red, scaly, or flakey; it may look smooth and shiny; or it may not look different at all.

Your baby may or may not have any symptoms of a yeast infection: Baby may or may not have white patches on his gums, cheeks, palate, tonsils, and/or tongue (if wiped off, they may look red or bleed). Baby may or may not have a diaper rash.

Because it is three times less likely that a yeast infection is the cause of breast pain, rule out other causes first, then see your health care provider for a diagnosis and treatment. See also "Get Checked for a Yeast Infection" in chapter 3 for more information.

If These Strategies Don't Work

If the information in this chapter has not reduced your breast pain, consider other possible causes:

- **Have you been setting your pump suction too high?** A pump suction that is too strong may cause temporary breast damage that can lead to pain. See the strategies for Problem 19.

- **Could you have mastitis?** For more, see Problem 13 in this chapter.

- **Does the breast pain start a minute or so into the feeding when baby starts gulping?** A very strong milk let-down can sometimes cause breast pain. This usually decreases and disappears during the first month of breastfeeding.

- **Do you lean over your baby in uncomfortable positions to breastfeed?** If so, try pillows or laid-back positions for better support.

- **Does the breast pain occur only during the days before your period?** If so, it may be related to hormonal changes and usually goes away after menstruation starts. If fibrocystic breast changes are a contributing factor, eliminating caffeine may help.

- **Are your breasts very large?** Large, heavy breasts can pull on the connective tissues above the breast, and you may feel tenderness where the breasts join the chest wall when you apply gentle pressure above your breasts. A different style or better-fitting bra may help relieve the pain.

Other, less common causes of breast pain include:

- **Pain from internal scarring from breast surgery or injury.** If the pain is severe, you can exclusively breastfeed from the other breast and avoid the painful one.

- **Pain from a ruptured breast implant.** In this case, you may see changes in breast shape or skin changes. See your health care provider if this is the case.

- **Pain from a milk-filled cyst called a** *galactocele.* With this harmless condition, you will usually feel an obvious lump in that breast.

The most important thing to remember is that breast pain is not a normal part of breastfeeding and that there is almost always a treatment or strategy that will make breastfeeding more comfortable. If you haven't yet found it in this chapter, it's time to seek skilled breastfeeding help. Don't settle for a painful experience. Get the help and support you deserve.

Chapter 5

Night Feedings

Lack of sleep and fatigue are a normal part of early parenthood, no matter how a baby is fed. This chapter includes realistic expectations and strategies that may put your situation into perspective, as well as help you get more rest.

Problem 15: Your newborn breastfeeds often at night and you feel exhausted.

During pregnancy, most parents know their newborns will wake at night to feed. But many are surprised at how often this happens. This section describes realistic expectations. It also provides time-tested strategies for getting more rest during your baby's early weeks and tips for shifting your newborn's longer sleep periods from day to night, where they belong.

Expect Topsy-Turvy Sleep Patterns

According to the typical newborn body clock, "night time is the right time," because most babies are born with their days and nights mixed up. Practically speaking, this means your baby will likely sleep more during the day and be more active (i.e., breastfeed like crazy) at night. Why are babies born this way? Maybe it's because during pregnancy babies are lulled to sleep during the day, when mothers are active, and are alert at night, when mothers lie still. But no one really knows for sure.

Understanding that these upside-down sleep-wake patterns are normal during the early weeks may ease your worries about your baby's nighttime feeding frenzies. Frequent night feedings do not mean your milk production is low or that you have a breastfeeding problem. That's just the way it is ... for now. But until it changes, you need some strategies for getting your rest. It may also help to keep in mind that, as with all things baby-related, this too shall pass.

Know What to Do If Baby Sleeps Longer Than Three Hours

Should you ever wake a sleeping baby? This depends. One four- to five-hour sleep stretch per day is in the normal range for a newborn. If your baby has one of these longer sleep stretches, thank your lucky stars! If you're really lucky, this longer stretch may happen at night. But don't count on it!

You don't need to wake your baby if her weight gain is good or if during the rest of each twenty-four-hour day she breastfeeds at least eight times. Many new parents are told to wake their babies at least every three hours, but that's not necessary, because what's actually important is the total number of daily feedings, not the time intervals between feedings. So in this case, if all other indicators look good, it's okay to let your baby sleep.

Nap While Baby Sleeps

Because you just had a baby, your body and mind need some downtime to adjust and recover. When your baby is active at night, napping during the day is the perfect solution. To make napping easier, be sure to accept all offers of help, especially from those who don't expect to be entertained and are happy to let you rest.

If you nap when your baby naps, it'll likely be at times when you would normally be awake and getting things done. But don't succumb to this temptation! If your baby is sleeping, stop worrying about writing thank-you notes, texting your friends, shopping, cleaning, surfing the Net, or making meals. Get on your baby's sleep rhythm and allow others to help you. This is not the time to be Superwoman. Make your rest a priority. You're worth it!

Tip: If baby keeps you awake at night, allow yourself to sleep during the day. Just like the total amount of mother's milk baby consumes in a twenty-four-hour period is key to her health, so are your cumulative hours of sleep. So rest when you can, even in short blocks of time.

Reset Your Baby's Body Clock

If your baby's internal clock says that midnight to 3 a.m. is party time, there are some tried-and-true strategies you can use to help her learn more quickly that nighttime is for sleeping.

After your milk increases on day 3 or 4, you can start helping baby to switch her longest sleep cycle from day to night. Keep in mind, though, it will probably take a few weeks to see significant changes. The main strategy here is to keep your usual nighttime sleeping hours as unstimulating for your baby as possible. How do you do that?

- **Keep the lights low.** Use just enough light to help see that your baby latches deeply. Turn on a nightlight, a lamp with its dimmer switch set on low, or a closet light with the door open a crack.

- **Keep it quiet.** Don't turn on your TV, tablet, or computer. Don't check your phone.

- **Change baby's diaper only when dirty.** Wait until morning to change wet diapers.

In other words, keep the night hours boring. Before you know it, your baby will realize that days are when the action happens, especially if during her daytime naps you keep her in well-lit areas with normal household noise.

After you've had a chance to rest and recuperate from birth, another way you can help baby reset her body clock is by interrupting any long sleep stretches during the day. After she's been sleeping for a couple of hours, wake her while she is in a light sleep (eyes moving under eyelids). This is not necessary from a breastfeeding standpoint, but it can help some babies more quickly shift their longer sleep stretch so it more closely matches yours.

Keep Baby Nearby at Night

To make night feedings less disruptive to your sleep, it helps tremendously for your baby to sleep near you. The less you have to move around at night to breastfeed, the easier it is for both of you to get back to sleep after feedings.

If anyone advises you against this, here's a great comeback: keeping baby close prevents sudden infant death syndrome (SIDS). This is why the American Academy of Pediatrics recommends that babies sleep in their parents' room for the first six months of life.

Options for keeping your baby close at night are amazingly varied, and every family comes up with its own variation. Some possibilities include:

- Baby sleeps in a bassinet next to your bed.

- Baby sleeps in a sidecar bed attached to yours.

- Baby sleeps in a crib with the side next to your bed removed and the crib pushed against your bed for easy access.

- Baby sleeps in a crib elsewhere in your room.

- Baby sleeps in your bed for all or part of the night (see "Make Your Sleep Surfaces Safe" later in this chapter).

- Baby (or you and baby together) sleep on a mattress (or a pallet, or a sleeping bag, etc.) on the floor in your room.

Myth: You'll get more sleep and feel more rested if someone else feeds the baby at night or if you give formula right before bedtime.

Reality: When mothers handle all night feedings they (and their partners) get more sleep than when night feedings are shared. In a 2007 study, Therese Doan and her colleagues compared the sleep patterns of first-time mothers and found that exclusively breastfeeding mothers get about forty-five minutes more sleep per night than their mixed-feeding or formula-feeding counterparts. In 2002 Diane Blyton and her colleagues found that exclusively breastfeeding mothers also spend more time in deeper sleep and feel less fatigued than those whose babies are fed formula.

Learn to Breastfeed Lying Down

Breastfeeding lying down is an incredible game-changer, because it allows you to sleep and feed at the same time. What a concept! Once you've mastered it, no one will have to sacrifice his or her rest to feed the baby.

Even if it takes you some practice to breastfeed in your sleep, don't give up! Breastfeeding lying down can be one of your best coping strategies in the early months. Once you've got it down pat, the issue of when your baby will sleep through the night loses much of its significance. It gets easier the more you do it and the older and more coordinated your baby becomes.

Practice When Awake

When you're first learning to breastfeed lying down, practice during your normal waking hours. Few of us learn best when we're half asleep. Once you get settled and your baby is breastfeeding, you can always take a nap. But start at a time when you feel awake and alert.

As you practice, the most important thing to keep in mind is that your own best way of breastfeeding lying down may be unique. How you feel most comfortable will depend on how you're made. Women have breasts of different sizes and shapes, arms of different lengths, and all sorts of body types. Be open to experimenting.

Start with a "V" Approach, Then Experiment with Other Positions

During the early weeks, side-lying feeding positions can be tricky, because gravity pulls your baby's body away from yours. Consider this approach a starting point. Then make adjustments to find your own best position.

1. Have within reach at least two pillows and a rolled-up hand towel or baby blanket.

2. Lie on your side, facing your baby, with a pillow under your head.

3. Put the other pillow behind your back.

4. Lay your baby completely on her side facing you, and align her body with yours so she is nose to nipple.

5. Pull her feet in close to you so your bodies form a V, which may be narrow or wide, depending on your breast size (see figure 5-1).

6. Lean back into the pillow behind your back until your nipple lifts off the bed, bringing it to the level of your baby's mouth.

7. Put the hand from your upper arm behind your baby's shoulders and pull her gently toward the breast, brushing her mouth and chin lightly against the breast until she opens wide.

8. Quickly move her onto the breast by pushing from behind her shoulders to help her get a good, deep latch.

9. Press her shoulders tightly against your body as she latches on.

10. Wedge the rolled-up towel or baby blanket behind her back to keep her in place, leaving her head free to angle back.

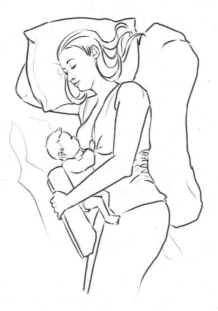

Figure 5-1. This mom and baby form a very narrow "V" when she pulls her feet in close.

©2012 Anna Mohrbacher, used with permission.

There are many different approaches to breastfeeding on your side, as you will see from the illustrations in this section. Try several until you find one you like. The V approach assumes your baby's head and body are resting on the bed, but some mothers prefer to rest their baby's head and body on their arm and use that arm to bring the baby onto the breast (see figure 5-2). If your baby spits up regularly, you may want to strategically position a bath towel under the two of you that you can easily roll up and replace as needed to avoid having to change sheets.

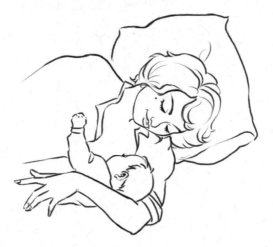

Figure 5-2. This mom supports her baby's head on her arm.

©2012 Anna Mohrbacher, used with permission.

There are also other ways. For example, mothers of twins often breastfeed at night resting on pillows propped up behind them, tucking a baby under each arm (see figure 5-3).

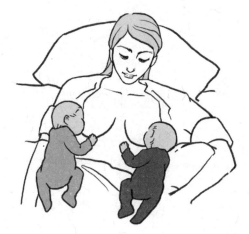

Figure 5-3. One way to breastfeed twins while lying down is with pillows for support.

©2012 Anna Mohrbacher, used with permission.

When it's time to switch breasts, you also have choices. You can pull your baby against your body, hold her against you while you roll over, and begin all over again on the other side. Or you can keep her where she is and lean over to feed from the upper breast (see figure 5-4). One thing's for sure, breastfeeding lying down is worth practicing until you can do it in your sleep.

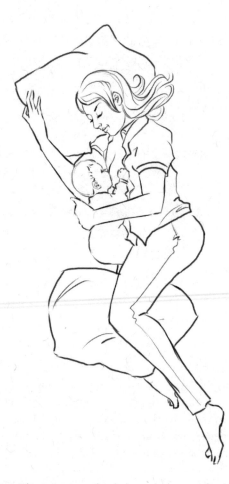

Figure 5-4. This mom props her baby on her arm to feed her from the upper breast.

©2012 Anna Mohrbacher, used with permission.

126

Some mothers worry about what to do about burping. Breastfed babies tend to take in much less air than babies who feed by bottle, so they may not need to be burped at all. You'll quickly get a sense of your own baby's needs. If your baby falls back asleep without burping, let her. She will wake and fuss if she needs to burp.

Make Your Sleep Surfaces Safe

There are safety standards for cribs and bedding when infants sleep alone, and there are also precautions that help keep babies safe when they sleep with their mother (see table 5-1). Breastfeeding mothers don't have to share a bed with their babies, but mothers lose less sleep and get more rest when they do. For this reason, many families sleep with their babies for at least part of the night. In some households, bedsharing is reserved for special occasions, illness, or naps. In others, parents and babies sleep together on a regular basis.

Critics of bedsharing warn that babies are at risk if they sleep somewhere other than a crib. The unfortunate and unintended effect of the "never bedshare" edict is that, when followed strictly, they inadvertently encourage far more dangerous nighttime behaviors. When a mother falls asleep while feeding on a sofa or recliner, for example, risk of infant death is sixty times greater than in an adult bed. Because the hormones of breastfeeding relax you, it is difficult to stay awake while breastfeeding at night, no matter where you are. In a 2010 survey of thousands of new mothers that was published in the journal *Clinical Lactation*, researcher Kathleen Kendall-Tackett and her colleagues noted that some mothers who fed their babies in upright positions at night even reported dropping their babies.

If you find that bedsharing works for you and your family, it is possible to make it safe. In Japan, for example, bedsharing is common, and the country's SIDS rates are among the lowest in the world. The typical Japanese family bed consists of a futon on the floor away from walls with nowhere for baby to fall or become wedged. Products are also available that can make an American adult bed safer, such as guardrails or large bolsters that make it impossible for babies to fall off.

The safe-sleep guidelines by the Academy of Breastfeeding Medicine (an association of physicians who support breastfeeding) in table 5-1 summarize how to achieve safe sleep in any sleep location and what unsafe sleeping practices to avoid. You can read this group's full statement with references at: www.bfmed. org/Media/Files/Protocols/Protocol_6.pdf.

If These Strategies Don't Work

If you've tried these strategies and are still feeling exhausted, don't despair. The good news is that this situation is temporary. As your baby grows and matures, developmental changes will also include changes in sleep patterns, eventually allowing you more precious hours for sleeping at night. As you try different sleeping arrangements, you will find one or more that lends itself to more rest at night, too.

Table 5-1. Guidelines Adapted from the Academy
of Breastfeeding Medicine

Safe sleeping practices

- Put baby on his back to sleep.

- Use a firm, flat surface, such as a firm mattress on the floor away from walls or a co-sleeping baby bed (sidecar) or crib that attaches to an adult bed.

- Tuck in any blankets around the mattress to avoid covering the baby's head.

- Dress baby in a warm sleeper if the room is cold.

Unsafe sleeping practices

- Exposing baby to smoke, either from you or secondhand smoke from others

- Sleeping with baby on a sofa, couch, daybed, or waterbed, or with pillows or loose bedding near baby

- Sleeping in a bed with an adjacent space that could trap baby

- Putting baby facedown or on his side for sleeping

- Sharing a bed with other children or an adult who is under the influence of alcohol, sedatives, or other mind-altering drugs

- Leaving baby alone on an adult bed

Problem 16: Your older baby or toddler still wakes often at night to breastfeed.

Many mothers are told that past a certain age (which varies by adviser) their breastfed babies don't *need* to breastfeed at night. However, in some cases, this simply isn't true. Read on to find out why.

Decide If Your Baby Needs to Breastfeed at Night

Due to individual differences among mothers and babies, some thriving breastfed babies sleep for long stretches at night early on, while others really do need to breastfeed at night—sometimes often—even at six months, eight months, ten months, and beyond. A mother's breast storage capacity is one individual difference that plays a major role in how often a baby needs to nurse, including during the night. Remember: it's not how much milk baby receives at each feeding, but rather how much milk he consumes in a twenty-four-hour day.

Breast storage capacity determines the number of milk removals needed each day (either by breastfeeding or pumping) to keep long-term milk production stable—and your baby healthy. Storage capacity is not related to breast size, but it does vary from woman to woman, which is why feeding patterns can vary so much among mothers—and why some babies *need* to breastfeed at night while another doesn't. After baby's first month, a mother with a large storage capacity will likely notice that her baby:

- Is satisfied with one breast at most or all feedings

- Is finished breastfeeding much sooner than other babies (maybe after just five to ten minutes)

- Gains weight well on fewer feedings per day than other babies.

- Sleeps for longer-than-average stretches at night

If this describes your breastfeeding experience, your baby may already be sleeping for longer stretches at night than other babies you know. But if after the first month of life your baby often takes both breasts at feedings, feeds on average longer than about ten to fifteen minutes total, typically takes eight or more feedings per day, and wakes more than once or twice a night to breastfeed, you likely have a small or average breast storage capacity.

It bears repeating that breastfed babies of both large- and small-capacity mothers receive plenty of milk. However, their breastfeeding patterns will by necessity differ in order for them to gain weight and thrive.

How does this apply to night feedings? A mother with a large storage capacity has the room in her breasts to comfortably store more milk at night before it exerts the amount of internal pressure needed to slow her milk production. On the other hand, if the baby of the small-capacity mother sleeps for too long at night, her breasts become so full that her milk production slows.

In other words, if you are a mother with an average or small breast storage capacity, night feedings may need to continue for many months for your milk production to stay stable and for your baby to thrive. Also, because your baby has access to less milk at each feeding, night feedings may be crucial for him to get enough milk overall. Again, what's important to a baby is not how much milk he receives at each individual feeding, but how much milk he consumes in a twenty-four-hour day. The good news is that you don't have to worry about this. If your baby has access to your breasts day and night and you nurse whenever he shows feeding cues, he will naturally stimulate and consume the right amount of milk. But it can be risky to mess with this reciprocal process. For example, if a mother with a small storage capacity uses *sleep training* strategies to force her baby to go for longer stretches between feedings, this may slow her milk production and compromise her baby's weight gain.

Sleep Norms Vary by Breast and Bottle

If you have a wakeful breastfeeding baby, one important question to ask yourself is: "Are my sleep expectations for my baby reasonable?" What you may be hearing from others about "normal" infant sleep may be based on research done on formula-fed babies who sleep in their own rooms. In general, breastfed babies are more wakeful and sleep for shorter stretches than formula-fed babies (the serious downside of longer sleep is that formula-fed babies are also at greater risk of SIDS than those breastfed). Another difference in sleep patterns is that breastfed six-month-olds typically wake as often as one-month-olds, so the expectation that the baby will sleep longer during the first six months of life does not appear to hold true.

Even into their second year, breastfeeding babies and toddlers do not conform to the expected sleep patterns of non-breastfed babies. For this reason, as breastfeeding becomes more common, expectations of babies' sleep patterns will need to change. In the meantime, however, many breastfeeding families regularly endure others' dismayed reactions to what is completely normal infant behavior and face social pressure from family, friends, and even health care providers to "correct" their "problem."

Myth: To prevent sleep problems, babies should learn to fall asleep on their own and never be allowed to fall asleep at the breast or in arms.

Reality: Babies have always fallen asleep at the breast, and the hormones of breastfeeding naturally encourage this. Although the idea of babies falling asleep on their own has become popular in recent decades, no research supports the long-term value of this strategy.

Reasons Babies Wake Other Than Hunger

Mothers often hope against hope that every time their baby sleeps a little longer for a while it means that their baby has outgrown night feedings. However, as any parent of older children will tell you, the only thing you can count on is that things will change.

When it comes to sleep, as babies grow there are many reasons why they wake at night and legitimately need your comfort, even when they're not hungry. This is just as true of formula-fed babies as it is of breastfed babies. Teething, which can last for many months, is one reason. If you've ever had a toothache as an adult, you know that you may not even notice it during the day when you're distracted by other things. But as soon as you lie down in bed, the throbbing and pain make it difficult to sleep. The same is true for babies. When teething pain

Myth: If you give your baby solid foods earlier than six months, he will sleep longer at night.

Reality: This popular belief has no basis in fact. Feeding solid foods does not result in longer sleep for babies. About the same number of babies begins sleeping more at night whether they receive solid foods or not. Sleeping longer at night is a developmental milestone that is unrelated to consumption of solid foods.

occurs, babies who had been sleeping longer may wake and want to nurse for comfort.

You don't need to worry about why your baby wants to nurse. Breastfeeding is an all-purpose mothering tool, and it's fine to use it to comfort your baby as well as to feed.

Entering a new stage of growth or development can also lead to frequent night-waking. Babies just learning to crawl, walk, or pull themselves up often become so fixated on their new skills that they begin practicing them unconsciously when in light sleep, which wakes them up.

Illness can also lead to frequent night-waking. Nursing a sick baby is not only a kindness—as breastfeeding is comforting—but more mother's milk at this time often leads to a faster recovery.

Have you ever laid in bed at night with your partner out of town and awoken feeling lonely? Babies can feel lonely, too. If you have a hard time sleeping alone, you can feel sympathy for babies who wake up feeling the same way. In many households, parents who would not dream of making their pets sleep alone think twice about responding to their baby's cries at night due to the dire warnings of the latest "sleep expert." But keep in mind that until about eighteen months of age, babies lack what's called *object permanence*, meaning that when you go away they are incapable of understanding that you'll come back. Reassuring your baby can do no harm because, despite what many say, the mental processes are not yet in place that allows him to manipulate you.

If you worry that your baby will have a lifetime of sleep problems unless you act now, recent studies and historical evidence on adult sleep suggest that sleeping through the night may not actually be normal for adults, either. To learn more, see: www. bbc.co.uk/news/magazine-16964783.

Reconsider Your Focus

In any healthy relationship, when there is a problem it makes sense to consider only those solutions that are respectful to both parties. If night feedings are normal and necessary for your breastfeeding baby, use coping strategies that respect both your need for sleep and your baby's need for milk. If you're sure your baby's night feedings are more of a *want* than a *need*, and you'd like to change this behavior, consider night-weaning options that are gradual and kind.

If you feel the need for another perspective, imagine you are five years in the future, reflecting back on this time. Would you feel pride or regret about how you handled your baby's sleep behaviors? Considering your long-term parenting goals may help you clarify your values and help you make choices along the way—even in the middle of the night. Also ask yourself whether you consider your baby's sleep behavior a problem for you or primarily a problem to others.

Adjust Your Sleeping Arrangements

To make night feedings less disruptive, it helps tremendously for your baby to sleep near you. The less you have to move around at night to breastfeed, the easier it is for both of you to get back to sleep after feedings. The advantage to this approach is that rather than focusing on trying to make your baby sleep for longer stretches at night (which may not be practical), you focus on those things you *can* control: maximizing your sleep while meeting your baby's need for milk.

There are many options for keeping your baby close by overnight. See "Keep Baby Nearby at Night" for examples. For ideas specific to a wakeful toddler, read on.

Create a Bedtime Routine

Elizabeth Pantley, whose *No-Cry Sleep Solution* book (see the Resources section) is a must-have authority on sleep matters, describes the advantages of structuring a peaceful bedtime routine that includes cuddling and focused time together so that your child can relax before sleeping. It also helps to structure your baby or toddler's environment so that the conditions that he awakens to in the night are the same that he experiences while going to sleep. For example, is the room temperature warm or cool? Are the windows and doors (to the closet, for example) open or shut? What noises can your baby hear? What level of light is in the room?

Tip: The more you can make your child's environment consistent at both bedtime and when he awakens at night, the easier it will be for him to go back to sleep.

Make Changes Gradually

Are you ready for a change in the nighttime routine? Is your baby? You might be ready to reduce night feedings, or you might have decided to give the family bed a try. Or maybe your partner wants to help with some nighttime feeding duties for a while.

Whether you decide to move your child's crib gradually farther and farther away from your bed, or you resolve to sleep with your child on a mattress on the floor in his room for a while before he is expected to sleep there by himself, take baby steps. Gradual change should get you there. And if it doesn't, try something else until it clicks.

Myth: Once you've begun a "bad habit" with a child, it will last a lifetime.

Reality: As long as a parent's expectations don't exceed the limits of his or her child's adaptability, most children respond well to gradual changes that are made with love.

If These Strategies Don't Work

If these suggestions don't bring about positive changes in your own sleep or your child's, there is most likely a reason. Perhaps the changes occurred too quickly or your child is truly not ready to take the next step. Or it may be time to schedule an appointment with your child's health care provider to rule out an allergy, reflux, or other conditions that could affect your child's sleep. Or maybe only time will tell.

You are not alone in your worries about sleep—yours or your baby's. However, know that your child will outgrow the babyish behavior you now find so concerning. It may also help to seek out other breastfeeding families and share experiences.

Chapter 6

Pumping

No one enjoys pumping, but you can make it a more pleasant experience by learning what to expect and how to maximize both your milk yields and your comfort. For many mothers, pumping is a key aspect of meeting their breastfeeding goals.

As this book explains, a pump can be a lifesaver if you're suffering from engorgement or nipple or breast pain. It allows many mothers to return to work while continuing to provide their milk to their babies. A little knowledge can go a long way in making your goal a reality.

Pumping can serve a useful purpose. However, it may cause anxiety when mothers second-guess their milk yields or worry about how long expressed milk can be safely stored. This chapter explores these topics and more.

Problem 17: You don't know which pump is right for you.

Many mothers are confused by the large variety of breast pumps on store shelves and on the Net. Choosing a pump is easier when you know which pumps are better suited for specific situations. Here are some examples.

Your Newborn Isn't Breastfeeding or Your Milk Supply Needs a Boost

In these situations, the recommended pump is the type mothers use while in the hospital. Some call these *hospital-grade* or *rental-grade breast pumps*. Another term is *multiuser pumps*, because when rented through hospitals, lactation consultants, pharmacies, and medical supply houses, the pump motor is shared among renters. But each mother buys her own milk-collection kit (the parts that come in contact with the milk), so one mother's milk never touches another's. A double milk-collection kit allows you to pump both breasts at the same time, which takes half the time of pumping one breast at a time with a single kit. These pumps are larger and heavier than those usually purchased for home or office use, because they are made to be durable enough to be used by many women.

These pumps do not provide stronger suction, as you don't want pump suction to be strong enough to cause skin damage. But most provide more choices of suction and speed settings and a smoother feel, making them a more effective substitute when a baby is not nursing at all or when a mother's milk production needs a boost.

You Are Returning to Work Full Time or Pumping Daily

In these situations, most mothers will get the best long-term results with a *professional-grade* double electric breast pump. Because they are not durable enough for sharing, professional-grade pumps are recommended for single-person use. Some brands of this type of pump are not safe to share because during use milk particles get sucked into the motor section and are blown back out, exposing baby to other mothers' milk. When shopping for this type of pump, check the motor warranty. Those with a motor warranty of one year or more will be less likely to break down with frequent use. These pumps come with a double milk-collection kit so pumping takes half the time of single pumping. Pumping time can be an important consideration in a work setting or if you're pumping often at home. Some models come with differing styles of carry bags, such as shoulder bags or backpacks, and some are available at lower prices without a carry bag. See the Resources section for links to the websites of several companies that make quality breast pumps.

You Work Part Time or Will Not Be Pumping Every Day

In these situations (especially if you work fewer than twenty hours per week), you probably will not be relying heavily on a breast pump to establish or maintain your milk production. This means you have many more pump choices. Keep in mind that if you buy a single pump, pumping one breast at a time takes twice as long as double pumping. A manual pump, which is usually powered by squeezing the pump's handle, can get tiring if you use it often. Visit some of the many websites that compare pump makes and models and choose those with the features most important to you.

Make Sure Your Pump Fits

Pump fit is not about breast size; it's about nipple size. It refers to how well your nipples fit into the pump opening or *nipple tunnel* (figure 6-1) that your nipple is pulled into during pumping.

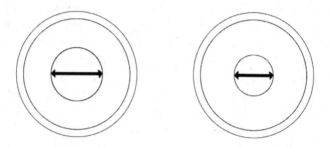

Figure 6-1. Pump nipple tunnels come in different sizes.

©2012 Anna Mohrbacher, used with permission.

You know you have a good pump fit if you see some (but not too much) space around your nipples as they move in and out of the nipple tunnel (figure 6-2). If your nipple rubs along the tunnel's sides, the tunnel is too small (figure 6-3). It can also be too large. Ideally, you want no more than about a quarter inch (6 mm) of the dark circle around your nipple (areola) pulled into the tunnel during pumping. If too much is pulled in, this can cause rubbing and soreness (figure 6-4). You'll know you need a different size if you feel discomfort during pumping even when your pump suction is near its lowest setting.

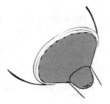

Figure 6-2. Some space around your nipple during pumping means you have a good fit.

©2012 Anna Mohrbacher, used with permission.

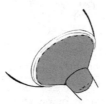

Figure 6-3. If your nipple rubs along the pump's tunnel, the tunnel is too small.

©2012 Anna Mohrbacher, used with permission.

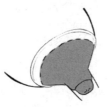

Figure 6-4. If too much areola is pulled in and rubs, the tunnel is too large.

©2012 Anna Mohrbacher, used with permission.

Don't assume that because you have large breasts, you'll need a large nipple tunnel. Small-breasted women can have large nipples and large-breasted women can have small nipples. Also, because few women are completely symmetrical, you may need one size nipple tunnel for one breast and another size for the other.

Getting a good fit is important, because your fit affects your pumping comfort and milk flow. If the nipple tunnel squeezes your nipple during pumping, this reduces your milk flow and you pump less milk. Also, either a too-large or too-small nipple tunnel can cause discomfort during pumping (see Problem 18).

Size Choices

When choosing a breast pump, find out if the brand you're considering offers multiple size options. If not, you're taking a chance. Most better breast pump companies sell a variety of nipple-tunnel sizes so that you can tailor your pump to your anatomy.

The popular Medela and Ameda brands offer six or seven size options and sell the part with the nipple tunnel separately, so you don't need to worry about buying the wrong size when you purchase these pumps. If you need another size, you can buy just that piece. The Medela nipple tunnels are also compatible with the Hygeia brand pumps. However, some breast pump brands, such as Avent and Evenflo, offer only two sizes. Their pumps are packaged with an insert piece that you can either leave in or remove. Other breast pump brands, such as Playtex, offer only one size.

Pump Fit Changes over Time

Once you find your best pump fit, it's not the end of the story. You need to recheck your fit every so often, because your nipples may expand with breastfeeding and pumping. In other words, although you see space around your nipples now, this space may eventually vanish. If your nipples begin to rub along your pump's nipple tunnel, don't be surprised. This just means it's time to switch to a larger nipple tunnel.

Problem 18: You think you should be pumping more milk.

Before deciding that your milk yield is too low, you first need to know what the average amount is for pumped milk. Many mothers discover—to their surprise—that when they compare their own pumping experience with the norm, they're doing just fine. Take a deep breath and read on.

Learn How Much Milk to Expect

If the first month of exclusive breastfeeding is going well, your milk production dramatically increases from about 1 ounce (30 mL) on day 1 to a peak of about 30 ounces (900 mL) per baby around day 40. Draining your breasts well and often naturally boosts your milk during these early weeks. But at first, while your milk production is ramping up, expect to pump less milk than you will later. If you remember pumping more milk for a previous child, you may be thinking back to a time when your milk production was already at its peak rather than during the early weeks while it was still building.

Prepare to Start Small

What should you expect when you begin pumping? First know that it takes time and practice to train your body to respond to your pump like it does to your baby. Don't assume (as many do) that what you pump is a gauge of your milk production. That is rarely the case, especially the first few times you pump.

It takes time to become proficient at pumping. Even with good milk production and a good-quality pump, some mothers find pumping tricky, especially at first. Be sure to give yourself enough time to learn to use your pump and to condition your body to its feel.

Think of your first pumping sessions as mostly practice, and don't expect to get much milk. Before you start seeing measurable amounts, you first need to train your body to respond to your pump as it does to your baby.

Know What Factors Can Affect Your Milk Yield

After you've had some practice using your pump, keep in mind that the following factors may affect your milk yield.

Your Baby's Age

How much milk a baby consumes per feeding varies by age and—until one month or so—by weight. Because newborns' stomachs are so small, during the first week most full-term babies take no more than 1 to 2 ounces (30 to 60 mL) at feedings. After about four to five weeks, babies reach their peak feeding volume of about 3 to 4 ounces (90 to 120 mL) of milk per session and 30 ounces per day (900 mL). (See table 2-1 for more average feeding volumes by age.)

Until your baby starts eating solid foods (recommended at around six months), her feeding volume and daily milk intake will not vary by much. Although a baby gets bigger and heavier between one and six months of age, her rate of growth slows down during that time, so the amount of milk she needs stays about the same. (This is not true for formula-fed babies.) Knowing this can be a huge relief if you are trying to keep up with your baby's need for milk after returning to work. When your baby starts eating solid foods, her milk demand will gradually decrease, as solids take your milk's place in her diet.

Whether or Not You Are Exclusively Breastfeeding

It's important to keep in mind that a mother who is exclusively breastfeeding her baby (offers no other liquids or solids to the child) and primarily does all of the feedings at the breast will yield more pumped milk than a mother giving formula regularly. This is because the milk production of the exclusively breastfeeding mother is greater, since her breasts are being drained more often and more fully.

Time Elapsed Since Your Last Milk Removal

On average, after an exclusively breastfeeding mother has practiced with her pump and it's working well for her, she can expect to pump:

- About half a feeding if she is pumping between regular feedings

- A full feeding if she is pumping for a missed feeding.

See table 2-1 "Baby's Average Feeding Volume by Age" for what a typical breastfeeding baby will ingest per feeding and per day. These averages will give you a sense of whether your pump yields are above average, below average, or right on. If you're giving formula and your baby is between one and six months old, you can calculate how much milk you should expect to pump at a session by determining what percentage of your baby's total daily intake is your milk. To do this, subtract from 30 ounces (900 mL) the amount of formula your baby receives each day. For example, if you're giving 15 ounces (450 mL) of formula each day, this is half of 30 ounces (900 mL), so you should expect to pump about half of what an exclusively breastfeeding mother would pump.

Time of Day

Most women pump more milk in the morning than later in the day. That's because milk production is not the same during the course of the day. To get the milk they need, many babies respond to this by simply breastfeeding more often when milk production is slower, usually in the afternoon and evening. Take advantage of this by pumping soon after you get up.

Tip: A good time to pump milk to store is usually thirty to sixty minutes after the first morning feeding. Most mothers will pump more milk then than at other times during the day.

Your Emotional State

Feeling upset, stressed, or angry releases adrenaline into your bloodstream, which inhibits your milk flow. For instance, if a mother of an ill preterm baby feels stressed after receiving bad news about her baby's condition, she will usually pump less milk. If you're experiencing negative feelings and aren't pumping as much milk as usual, take a break and pump later, when you're feeling calmer and more relaxed.

Your Breast Storage Capacity

This is the maximum amount of milk available in your breasts during the time of day when your breasts are at their fullest. Storage capacity is based on the amount of room in your milk-making glands, not breast size. It varies among mothers and in the same mother from baby to baby. Mothers with a large storage capacity usually pump more milk at a session than mothers with a small storage capacity. Want to find out what your capacity is? If you're exclusively breastfeeding your baby and pumping for a missed feeding, a milk yield (from both breasts) of much more than about 4 ounces (120 mL) may indicate a larger-than-average storage capacity. On the other hand, if you never pump more than 3 ounces (90 mL), even when it has been many hours since your last milk removal, your storage capacity may be smaller than average.

What matters to your baby is not how much she gets at each feeding, but how much milk she receives during a twenty-four-hour day. Breast storage capacity explains many of the differences in breastfeeding patterns and pump yields that are common among mothers. See "Keep an Eye on Your Magic Number" in chapter 2 for more information on breast fullness and breast storage capacity.

Pump Performance and Suction Setting

First make sure you've chosen the best pump for your situation—and that it's a good fit—by reading the strategies in Problem 17. Next, check the suction setting. Common sense might tell you that a stronger pump suction should yield more milk. But, in this case, common sense is wrong. At too-high suction settings, you may actually pump less milk. That's because tensing up from discomfort can inhibit your milk flow. (If you're gritting your teeth or your nipples are sore afterward, it's too high!) If you set your pump suction too low or too high, you'll likely get less milk.

Myth: To get more milk, set your pump suction to the highest setting.

Reality: Your most effective suction setting may be well below your pump's maximum. To get the most milk, set your pump to the highest suction setting that's truly comfortable for you.

How do you find your best setting? Turn up your pump suction until it feels slightly uncomfortable and then turn it down slowly. Stop when you reach the highest setting that feels *completely comfortable* to you. You may end up on your pump's maximum setting, minimum setting, or anywhere in between. The maximum comfortable suction setting is what you're striving for, not a specific place on your pump's controls.

Trigger More Milk Releases

The key to pumping more milk is not stronger suction but more *let-downs*, or milk releases. The fewer milk releases triggered during pumping, the less milk pumped. With no milk release, you'll express only the small amount of milk pooled around your nipples, at most about half an ounce (15 mL) per breast.

What is a milk release? It's when the muscles inside the breast squeeze the milk-making glands and push the milk out of the breast. Without it, most of the milk stays in your breast. Milk release is caused by the hormone oxytocin. Some mothers feel it as a tingling sensation or see it as leaking milk; others feel and see nothing. By watching your milk flow during pumping, you will see your milk releases as an obviously faster milk flow. During breastfeeding, you can hear milk releases when your baby begins gulping.

Most mothers average about five let-downs at each breastfeeding without even realizing it. Some perceive the first milk release as a pins-and-needles sensation or cramping in their breasts, but very few feel the later milk releases. Some mothers feel none. Even if you don't feel a milk release, your baby's swallowing tells you they're happening. And your baby's weight gain is sure proof that breastfeeding is working as it should.

While your baby is at the breast, milk release is triggered by her suckling, the feel of her soft skin against yours, her warmth, and your loving thoughts. Even when baby is not breastfeeding, a milk release can happen when your breasts are touched, you hear your baby (or another baby) cry, even when you think about your baby. Feelings of tension, anger, or frustration can block it.

When you pump, your baby's softness and warmth are missing. Suction from a piece of plastic feels very different from your baby's warm mouth and tongue movements. As you train your body to respond to the feel of the pump, you may need extra help to trigger let-downs. You may also need extra help when you switch from one pump to another, because the new pump has a different feel than your former pump.

Use Your Senses to Trigger Milk Releases

If you need help to release your milk to the pump, try the following suggestions, which incorporate different types of sensory stimulation.

- **Feelings:** Get comfortable, and pump in a private space where you can relax. Close your eyes and imagine your baby at the breast. Breathe deeply and think about how much you love your baby. Imagine yourself in a tranquil, relaxed place.

- **Sight:** Look at your baby or a photo of her. Or play a video of her.

- **Hearing:** Play a recording of your baby cooing or crying. Call to check on your baby, or call someone you love to relax and distract you.

- **Smell:** Smell your baby's blanket or clothing while you pump.

- **Touch:** Gently massage your breasts or apply warm compresses.

- **Taste:** Sip a favorite warm drink to relax you.

You may only need to use one or two of these strategies for a short time until you condition your body to respond to the feel of your pump.

Vary Your Pump Speed

Most babies suckle more rapidly at first to trigger a milk release and then use slower jaw movements while the milk is flowing to drain the breast. If your pump has a speed or cycle control, you can mimic your baby's rhythm to get more milk more quickly.

1. Start pumping on the "fast" setting.

2. Go to a "slow" setting when milk starts flowing.

3. Return to a "fast" setting after milk flow slows.

4. Repeat until you see at least three to five milk releases.

If you have a two-phase pump with a let-down button, be aware that these pumps are programmed to automatically switch from a fast to slow speed after two minutes of pumping, because that's how long it takes on average for a let-down to occur. If your body takes more or less time to let down your milk, you can customize the pump to work better for you by depressing this button for a faster speed whenever your milk flow slows and pushing it again to go to a slower speed when the next let-down occurs. You can use the let-down button several times during the pumping to speed up the milk-removal process. Your baby would do this automatically, but you can mimic this pattern by adjusting your pump according to your milk flow.

Try Hands-On Pumping

Until 2009, most mothers assumed that their pump should do all of the milk-removal work. But this changed when Jane Morton and her colleagues published a groundbreaking study in the *Journal of Perinatology*. The mothers in this study were pumping exclusively for premature babies in the hospital's neonatal intensive care unit. For premature babies, mother's milk is like a medicine. Because receiving any infant formula increases their risk of serious illness, these mothers were under a lot of pressure to pump enough milk to meet their babies' needs.

Amazingly, when these mothers used their hands as well as their pump to express milk, they pumped an average of 48 percent more milk than the pump alone could remove. Rather than their milk production faltering after three to four weeks of pumping, which was common for many mothers of premature babies, the mothers using this "hands-on" technique continued to increase their milk production throughout their babies' entire first eight weeks.

Hands-on pumping is not just for mothers with babies in special care. Any mother who does a lot of pumping can benefit from it. How does it work? Follow these steps:

1. First, massage both breasts.

2. Double-pump (pump both breasts at the same time), compressing your breasts often while pumping. Continue until milk flow slows to a trickle.

3. Massage your breasts again, concentrating on any areas that feel full.

4. Finish by either hand-expressing your milk into the pump's nipple tunnel or by single-pumping, whichever yields the most milk. Either way, during this step, do intensive breast compression on each breast, moving back and forth from breast to breast several times until you've drained both breasts as fully as possible.

This entire routine took the mothers in the study an average of about 25 minutes. Online videos demonstrate this technique. See "How to Use Your Hands When You Pump" at: newborns. stanford.edu/Breastfeeding/MaxProduction.html. The following two online videos demonstrate two different hand-expression techniques that can be used as part of hands-on pumping: newborns.stanford.edu/Breastfeeding/HandExpression.html and ammehjelpen.no/handmelking?id=907 (scroll down for the English version).

Hands-on pumping can be used by any mother who wants to improve her pumping milk yield or boost her milk production. It works because hands-on pumping helps drains your breasts more fully—and drained breasts make milk faster.

Expect Baby to Take More Milk When Bottle-Fed

If your baby consumes more milk from the bottle than you can pump at one sitting, does this mean your milk production is low? Not necessarily. Even if you're pumping at a time you'd usually be breastfeeding, this may not be the case. Why?

Milk Intake Differs by Feeding Method

Have you ever been told to eat slowly so that your *appetite-control mechanism* takes effect? Eating too fast can lead to overeating, because it takes time for your body to realize you've had enough. By eating more slowly, you will feel full after eating less food. The same is true for babies.

Milk suckled from the breast has a natural ebb and flow. During breastfeeding, after each milk release ends there is usually a short time when milk flow slows to a trickle. As explained before, the cycle repeats an average of five times during each breastfeeding. The ebb and flow allows baby's appetite-control mechanism to take effect, leaving her full on less milk.

When you feed your baby by bottle—whether it contains your milk or formula—its consistently fast flow can result in your baby eating more after she's had enough milk. This is because her appetite-control mechanism hasn't signaled fullness to her brain yet. It's also one reason bottlefeeding puts babies at increased risk for obesity later in life.

Tip: If your baby is taking more milk from the bottle than you are pumping, this may simply be a reflection of the differences in milk-delivery system, not a sign of low milk production. At the breast babies older than one month old take on average 3 to 4 ounces (90 to 120 mL) of milk; those same babies often take much more than this from the bottle.

The most reliable way to know if you're producing the milk your baby needs is her weight gain. For instance, if during the first three to four months your baby is exclusively fed your milk and gaining an average of 1 ounce per day, you have nothing to worry about.

If These Strategies Don't Work

Breast pumps work well for the vast majority of women, but there are exceptions. If you have tried all the suggestions in this section yet still find that you are unable to pump your milk effectively, one option is to switch from a personal pump to a hospital-grade rental pump. Some mothers get better results with these types of pumps.

Another alternative is a time-tested approach commonly used in other parts of the world: hand expression. There are many ways to hand express milk. See the Resources section for a list of instructional videos.

Problem 19: Pumping is painful.

Some mothers assume pumping should be painful. Not so! "No pain, no gain" does not apply here. Painful pumping means something needs to be adjusted. What causes pain? The two most common causes are: 1) pump suction set too high, and 2) pump fit problems.

Lower Your Pump's Suction

Pumping milk is not like drinking from a straw. With a straw, the stronger you suck, the faster the liquid flows. When pumping, most milk comes only when a *let-down*, or milk release, happens. Many factors affect when a milk release occurs and some can inhibit it, including a suction setting that is too high. See "Pump Performance and Suction Setting" earlier in this chapter to achieve the right pump setting for you.

Check Your Pump Fit

Fit refers to the size of the opening your nipple is drawn into during pumping, otherwise known as the *nipple tunnel* (see figure 6-1). Many mothers pump comfortably with the standard size that comes with their pump. But if pumping hurts even on low suction, you most likely need a larger- or smaller-sized opening. A better-fitting nipple tunnel will feel more comfortable and may even pump more milk. See "Make Sure Your Pump Fits" earlier in this chapter to determine if your pump is a good match for you.

If These Strategies Don't Work

If you've ruled out a pump suction that is too strong and fit problems as the cause of your painful pumping, here are more strategies to consider.

Try Soft Inserts

Some women find pumping uncomfortable when their breasts are pulled against hard plastic. If you don't have an Avent or Playtex pump, which comes with a soft silicone insert, you can buy them separately and try them with your pump. Soft insert options include the Avent Isis Petal Massager and the Ameda Flexishield Areola Stimulator (see the Resources section for websites).

Note that the Ameda version narrows your nipple tunnel to its smallest size (21 mm), so this option won't be a good choice if you need a larger nipple tunnel size.

Check Your Nipple and Breast Health

Sometimes pain during pumping can occur when your breasts or nipples are tender from other causes. To consider this possibility, answer the following questions.

- Do you have broken skin on one or both of your nipples? If you have previously had nipple trauma, could you have developed a bacterial infection of the nipple? Might you have an overgrowth of yeast, also known as *thrush* or *candida*? If the answer to any of these questions is yes, see chapter 3.

- Do you have a tender or painful area or lump in your breast? Does your nipple turn white, red, or blue after pumping? If your answer is yes to either of these questions, see chapter 4.

If a nipple- or breast-related health issue may be the cause of your painful pumping, see an international board-certified lactation consultant or other health care provider to evaluate you for possible treatment.

Problem 20: You don't know which milk-storage guidelines to follow.

Reading different milk-storage guidelines in different places can be confusing and even upsetting. Why can't the experts agree among themselves? What guidelines should you follow? To find out, read on.

Understand Why Guidelines Differ

You'll notice that some of the milk-storage times in table 6-2 are labeled "Okay" while others are labeled "Ideal." Within the "Okay" times, pumped milk should not spoil. As time passes, however, even though the milk is still "good," more vitamins, antioxidants, and immunological factors are lost. The shorter storage times labeled "Ideal" correspond to the guidelines some organizations advise because fewer of these factors are lost.

The bottom line is that while it is always better to use your milk sooner rather than later, your milk should not spoil if you store it within the timeframe marked "Okay." Stored milk that you find in the back of the fridge that has been there for up to eight days will still be far better for your baby than formula.

Some milk-storage guidelines also vary because they define "room temperature" differently. If you live in a subtropical climate, for example, the higher room-temperature range in table 6-2 may better fit your reality. But if you live in the frigid north, the lower range may better fit yours.

You may also notice that refrigerator storage times for fresh and refrigerated milk are longer than those for previously frozen milk. This difference is because freezing kills the antibodies in the milk, making the milk more susceptible to spoilage. When in doubt about the freshness of your milk, smell or taste it. Spoiled milk will smell spoiled.

Table 6-2. Milk Storage Times for Full-Term Healthy Babies at Home

Milk Storage/ Handling	Deep Freezer (0°F/-18°C)	Refrigerator Freezer (variable 0°F/-18°C)	Refrigerator (39°F/4°C)	Insulated Cooler with Ice Packs (59°F/15°C)	Room Temperature (66°F–72°F/ 19°C–22°C)	(73°F–77°F/ 23°C–25°C)
Fresh	Ideal: 6 months Okay: 12 months	3–4 months	Ideal: 72 hours Okay: 8 days	24 hours	6–10 hours	4 hours
Frozen, thawed in fridge	Do not refreeze	Do not refreeze	24 hours	Do not store	4 hours	4 hours
Thawed, warmed, not fed	Do not refreeze	Do not refreeze	4 hours	Do not store	Until feeding ends	Until feeding ends
Warmed, fed	Discard	Discard	Discard	Discard	Until feeding ends	Until feeding ends

Use Your Situation as a Guide

If you're still in doubt about which milk-storage guidelines to follow and the best way to store your milk, ask yourself the following questions.

- **Is your baby healthy?** The guidelines in table 6-2 are intended for full-term, healthy babies at home. If your baby is hospitalized, the milk-storage guidelines your hospital gives you are likely to be shorter than these. Because premature and sick babies are at higher risk for serious health problems, they may also recommend you use stricter hygiene than you will need to follow later, such as storing your milk in sterile containers or boiling your pump parts regularly.

- **How much pumped milk does your baby get?** If your baby gets most of his milk directly from the breast, you don't need to worry about whether the relatively small amount of pumped milk he gets is fresh, refrigerated, or previously frozen. However, if a substantial percentage of your baby's daily milk intake is expressed milk, consider more carefully your milk-storage choices. For example, because freezing kills the antibodies in the milk, which help keep baby healthy, rather than freezing all of your pumped milk, feed your baby as much fresh or refrigerated milk as possible. Also keep in mind that even without the antibodies, frozen milk is still a far healthier choice than formula.

Chapter 7

Weaning

Sooner or later every breastfeeding baby weans from the breast. Despite how commonplace weaning is, it can be fraught with doubts, misconceptions, and worries. Is baby weaning too soon? Can you breastfeed too long? Is pain from engorged breasts inevitable? Can you make weaning a positive experience, even when your toddler resists your efforts? Read on for answers to these questions and more.

Problem 21: You're unsure whether to wean now or later.

Before children, breastfeeding decisions can seem so simple. After children, their complexities come into focus. Motherhood changes us, and even if you started breastfeeding with a clear end date in mind, when that time comes you may have doubts about stopping. Or circumstances may cause you to question whether making it to your goal is realistic.

Review Your Goals and the Experts' Recommendations

Did you start breastfeeding with a goal of six weeks, three months, six months, one year, two years, longer? Every family has its own ideas about when to wean and its own unique considerations that influence this decision. If you are rethinking your personal goals, it may help to start with what the experts say about how long to breastfeed and why.

What the Experts Say

In 2012, the American Academy of Pediatrics (AAP), the organization that educates pediatricians on best medical practices, updated its policy statement on breastfeeding. In 2005, it recommended a minimum of one year of breastfeeding. After reviewing the research published since then, it reached the same conclusion.

Why did the AAP's expert panel recommend breastfeeding for at least the first year of life? In short, because according to the science, the short- and long-term health of both mother and child are measurably worse when breastfeeding ends earlier than this.

- **Breastfeeding for at least one year is important to your baby's health.** When your baby weans before one year, this puts her at greater risk of catching many illnesses of infancy, including colds, ear infections, diarrhea, and more serious diseases like meningitis, bronchitis and pneumonia. But the health effects of breastfeeding extend far beyond babyhood. Weaning before age one also increases her risk later in life of becoming obese and developing health problems such as asthma, allergies, diabetes, celiac disease, childhood cancers, leukemia, and inflammatory bowel diseases.

- **Breastfeeding for at least one year is important to the mother's health, too.** Your weaning decision affects your long-term health as well. There is a common misconception that breastfeeding is a drain on a mother's health and energy, but science tells us the opposite is true. While a mother breastfeeds, despite what many think, she sleeps longer and deeper (for more on this see "Keep Baby Nearby at Night" in chapter 5) and her metabolism is more efficient than after weaning. In general, the longer and more exclusively you breastfeed your baby, and the more months total you breastfeed during your lifetime, the better for your health. Even decades after your baby weans, breastfeeding for less than a year increases your risk of developing breast and ovarian cancers, rheumatoid arthritis,

Myth: Most experts recommend weaning by one year of age.

Reality: One year is the *minimum* age of weaning—not the maximum age of breastfeeding—recommended by the American Academy of Pediatrics. The World Health Organization recommends at least two years of breastfeeding. Both groups—and many others—encourage mothers and babies to continue breastfeeding as long after this minimum age as mutually desired. From a health perspective, the longer you breastfeed, the better.

type 2 diabetes, and cardiovascular disease, the number-one killer of women.

Even into a child's second and third year of life, scientists have found that weaned children are more likely to become ill and even die than children who are still breastfeeding. The living antibodies in human milk work their magic for as long as your child is at the breast. The same is true for you. The longer you breastfeed, the lower your risk of many serious health problems.

What If Your Baby Decides to Wean Before One Year?

Sometimes weaning before one year seems to be the baby's idea. However, if a baby younger than one appears to be weaning, it is more likely to be a *nursing strike*, because a baby this age still has a physical need for mother's milk. A nursing strike is when a baby who was breastfeeding well suddenly refuses the breast. Another clue that this "decision" may not be a natural weaning is that the baby is usually unhappy about it. See Problem 3 for strategies to overcoming a nursing strike and bringing baby back to breastfeeding. This may require some ingenuity, but it can be done.

Can You Breastfeed Too Long?

You may have noticed that both the AAP and the World Health Organization (WHO) recommend a minimum period of breastfeeding but say nothing about how long is too long. Why is this? There are two main reasons. First, these organizations know that from a health perspective the longer you breastfeed your child, the better. Whether your breastfeeding child is two, three, four, or even older, the living components of your milk contribute to her good health. Second, the experts know that even if you make no attempt to wean, your baby will eventually outgrow breastfeeding and stop on her own. That's why the AAP's 2012 statement leaves its recommendation open-ended by saying that after one year breastfeeding should continue as long thereafter as mutually desired.

At what age do children outgrow breastfeeding? Learning more about weaning practices in other times and places may answer this question and give you a broader perspective on your options. Some mothers wean before they feel ready because others convince them that they are being "selfish" or harming their child by breastfeeding past a certain age. But what our culture considers normal is at the very early end of the broader human experience. Knowing this can give you more freedom to make your own decisions rather than being unduly swayed by others.

When human cultures are viewed as a whole, the average age of weaning is between two and four years, with some societies breastfeeding for as long as five to seven years. History tells us that breastfeeding for years was common practice in most times and places, including in the colonial United States. Interestingly, most religions' holy books address the age of weaning. The Koran recommends breastfeeding for at least two years, the Torah three years, and Hindu Ayurvedic texts two to three years. Does this mean you should breastfeed this long? Not necessarily. But if you decide to breastfeed longer than most people you know, you can rest assured that this is not harmful to either you or your child.

Decide If Weaning Is the Best Option

Many women think first of weaning when they find themselves in the situations described below. Weaning for these reasons may seem like an obvious choice, but before starting this process, read on and decide if weaning is indeed your best option.

You Have an Unresolved Breastfeeding Problem

If you haven't yet sought skilled breastfeeding help, now is the time. You may believe your situation is hopeless, but before weaning, seek help from an international board-certified lactation consultant. Her job is to know all the strategies you haven't yet tried. The vast majority of breastfeeding problems are fixable.

You're Returning to Work

Many women successfully combine breastfeeding and working. But even if you can't pump at work, you can still breastfeed when you're home. By gradually reducing your milk production to a lower level (see "Wean Gradually" in this chapter), you can comfortably go for long stretches without needing to pump. Some breastfeeding is always better than none.

A Health Care Provider Told You to Wean

Not all health care providers are knowledgeable about breastfeeding. If a health care provider recommends weaning, get a second opinion, and discuss it with a lactation consultant.

You Need to Take Medication

Most drugs are compatible with breastfeeding, which means that the risks of giving formula is considered greater than the risks of taking the drug while continuing to breastfeed. If you want information about whether a drug is compatible with breastfeeding, call the Infant Risk Center at 806-352-2519. Its experts are available Monday through Friday from 8 a.m. to 5 p.m. (CST). You can also check with a lactation consultant about the safety of a prescription or over-the-counter drug.

You or Your Baby Is Ill or Hospitalized

This is usually the worst time to wean, as an ill baby will almost always recover faster if breastfeeding continues. And the last thing an ill or injured mother needs is the added pain and health risks of an abrupt weaning. If weaning is absolutely necessary, see "Wean Gradually" in this chapter for strategies for making the transition comfortable. Remember: you can also use a breast pump to wean gradually if your baby can't breastfeed.

You Are Pregnant

Some women choose to wean during pregnancy, but you don't have to. There is no evidence that breastfeeding is harmful in any way to you or your unborn baby, unless your pregnancy is so high risk that you are told to abstain from sex, which releases the same hormones as breastfeeding.

Your Baby Has Teeth

In most places around the world, babies breastfeed long past the age of teething. If your baby is biting (most don't), see Problem 11 for ways to stop the biting without weaning.

You Feel Overwhelmed with Breastfeeding

If this is your reason for weaning, consider seeking skilled breastfeeding help. Someone who can work with you in person, hands on, is a valuable supplement to the strategies in this book. Think also about why you feel this way. For example, some mothers with a history of childhood sexual abuse find the intimate contact of breastfeeding difficult, even when it's going well. In this case, you still have options. For example, you may pump your milk and bottlefeed it to baby for some or all feedings. You may also do a partial weaning, eliminating some regular breastfeedings until you feel more at ease. Some breastfeeding is always better than none.

Others Are Pressuring You to Wean

It takes a strong person to continue breastfeeding in spite of an unsupportive partner, family, or social circle. If this is your situation, look for the support you need elsewhere, such as weekly hospital mothers' meetings, drop-in breastfeeding cafés, or online or in-person mother-to-mother breastfeeding gatherings. Meeting with other like-minded women—even once in a while—can make a tremendous difference. See the Resources section for details.

Determine If Your Expectations for Weaning Are Realistic

Some mothers consider weaning in the hopes that it will improve other aspects of their own or their baby's life in some way. What follows are a few common "aspirations" mothers have that they believe can be achieved through weaning. It might work in your case, but typically weaning is not the solution in these situations, and ending breastfeeding can backfire in unexpected ways.

Your Baby Will Sleep Longer at Night

Not always. Some mothers wean newborns to formula for this reason, only to discover after weaning that their sleep patterns are unchanged and now night feedings require a wide-awake adult.

Your Toddler Will Be More Independent

Mothers of toddlers sometimes wean for this reason only to find that their child becomes clingier. Independence is unrelated to breastfeeding and occurs naturally over time and growth with a secure emotional attachment.

Weaning Will Make Your Life Easier

This is an admirable goal, but sometimes life can actually become more challenging after weaning. For example, if your child wakes at night, after weaning it may require more effort on your part to settle her down. She is likely to get sick more often—which may mean taking more time off work. And you will lose the calming and comforting mothering tool of breastfeeding.

Recognize the Right Time to Wean

If you're feeling doubts about weaning, consider this a sign that the time may not be right. You'll know your time has come when you have all the facts, know all your options, and you (or your baby) make the decision to wean. Here are some indicators that your time to wean has come.

You Feel Ready

You've met your breastfeeding goals or have decided to wean based on your own unique considerations. It is clear to you that the time is right.

Your Child Is Ready

Even if you do nothing to wean your child, all children will eventually outgrow breastfeeding, sometimes even before you feel ready to wean. If your child is older than one year, she may indeed be ready to make this major transition.

You Have a Confirmed Medical Issue

"Confirmed" means you've gotten a second opinion, as well as spoken to a lactation consultant. Medically valid reasons to wean involving your health are rare. Examples include chemotherapy to treat cancer and radioactive therapy for thyroid problems.

Tip: If, after giving all the strategies in this section a try, you're still feeling unsure about weaning, consider this a sign you are probably not ready to end breastfeeding. Maybe you'll feel differently next week, next month, or next year. If for now you have serious doubts, listen to your inner voice. Trust your instincts.

Problem 22: Your breasts hurt during weaning.

It's not uncommon for breasts to feel full or uncomfortable during the weaning process, especially after dropping a feeding. Discomfort or pain is usually a sign you may be weaning too quickly. Take it in baby steps, and use a pump when needed to make the process more comfortable for you.

Wean Gradually

Slowing down the weaning process may be all you need to relieve your breast pain. But the devil is in the details.

For the baby younger than one year, infant formula is the recommended substitute for mother's milk. (Straight cow's milk is okay after one year.) Your baby's age will help you determine how to feed it to him. If your baby is nine months to a year old and drinking well from a cup, you can skip the bottle entirely, which avoids the need to wean again from a bottle later.

Here's how to make a gradual weaning happen step-by-step:

- First, take note of the times each day you usually breastfeed.

- Pick one daily breastfeeding (reserve the first morning breastfeeding for last) and instead feed your baby infant formula by bottle or by cup, if he's mastered it.

- Give your body at least two to three days to adjust to the decreased demand before dropping another daily breast-feeding. This way your milk production can be reduced comfortably and gradually.

Following this plan, it usually takes about two to three weeks to go from exclusive breastfeeding to a complete weaning. A gradual weaning like this is not just more comfortable and safer for you. It is also good for your baby because you have time to make sure he is handling infant formula well before your milk is gone. It also gives you time to help your baby adjust to this change by giving him extra attention as a substitute for the closeness you shared at the breast.

Pump to Comfort

As you follow the steps to wean gradually, you may notice that your breasts begin to feel full. In this instance, don't hesitate to *pump to comfort*. This means pumping just enough milk to relieve your breast fullness and no more.

Some mothers hesitate to do this because they worry it will stimulate more milk production and take them in the wrong direction. In reality, pumping to comfort is the best thing you can do, because it allows your milk production to decrease gradually enough to prevent two problems you don't need: breast pain, which can become severe, and breast infection, also known as *mastitis*, a condition that can be caused by lengthy and unrelieved breast fullness (see chapter 4). Pay attention to your body's cues and pump to comfort whenever you feel the need.

If These Strategies Don't Work

If your breast pain is severe and continues despite the suggestions above, you may have developed an inflammation or infection in the breast. See Problem 13 for resolution.

Problem 23: Your toddler resists weaning.

The child older than one year usually has strong preferences about breastfeeding, along with all other aspects of her routine. Even so, it's possible with a little foresight and planning to make weaning a positive experience. To accomplish this, first allow enough time so you aren't rushing the process. If your child is breastfeeding often, for example, you may need several weeks to wean; for each daily breastfeeding you eliminate, you need to allow your body two to three days to comfortably reduce your milk production before you eliminate the next feeding.

To keep your weaning positive, as you proceed respect your toddler's temperament and preferences. Think about foods, drinks, and activities she might consider even better than breastfeeding, and offer them as much as possible. Also, certain nursings may be more important to her than others. If so, allow your child to give them up last. (Often the bedtime breastfeeding is a favorite.) Consider each of the following strategies in light of what you know about your own child. Use those that work and pass on those that don't.

Don't Offer, Don't Refuse

This means breastfeed when your baby asks, and don't offer the breast when she doesn't ask. When used in combination with the following strategies, this can speed up the weaning process.

Tip: Children often ask to breastfeed when they're hungry or thirsty. Eliminate this reason to breastfeed by keeping your toddler's hunger and thirst at bay with regular meals, snacks, and drinks.

Plan Interesting Activities

Breastfeeding may not even enter your child's mind if you offer age-appropriate and fun alternatives to nursing that keep her happily busy in other ways. This will prevent her from asking to breastfeed out of boredom.

Change Your Routine

Think about the times and places your child asks to breastfeed. Then consider how to change your routine so she will be reminded of nursing less often. For example, if she usually asks to breastfeed when you sit in a certain chair, avoid that chair for now. If she nurses to sleep at naptime and she's ready to give up a nap, make that change in routine to eliminate that feeding.

Get Your Partner Involved

Sleep-related nursings can be the trickiest to eliminate without a fuss, such as when your child breastfeeds to go to sleep, while half asleep, or just after waking up. This is when your partner can be a huge help. To eliminate that first morning breastfeeding, ask your partner to help your child get up for the day and give her breakfast. Your partner can also develop new going-to-bed routines and help her get back to sleep when she wakes at night. But don't restrict your partner's help to nights and mornings. During the day your partner can also help keep weaning positive by planning special daytime outings together to distract her from her usual routine.

Before Baby Asks, Offer Substitutes and Distractions

Offering alternatives to the breast before your child asks to breastfeed is important to a positive weaning, because once she's asked to nurse she may get upset if you offer a substitute. One way to do this is to offer a special snack and drink right before a usual breastfeeding time, and then take her to a favorite place, such as a playground, as a distraction. Some children breastfeed more often at home with nothing to do and less often when out and distracted. For this type of child, spend as much of the day as possible out of the house. On the other hand, if your child breastfeeds more often when she's in new surroundings, stay home more and keep distractions to a minimum.

Postpone

Postponing breastfeeding can work well for a child who nurses at irregular times and places and is old enough to accept waiting (maybe age two or three). On the other hand, if postponing leaves your child feeling as though you are keeping her at arm's length, she may become even more determined to breastfeed. If so, other strategies will be better.

Shorten Your Breastfeeding Time

Restricting breastfeeding to a shorter time is most effective with children older than two and can be a good start to the weaning process. Some mothers use this as an introduction to clocks and time, and have their toddlers help them determine when their time at breast is done.

Bargain

An older child who is close to outgrowing breastfeeding may give up breastfeeding earlier by mutual agreement. But most children younger than three do not have the maturity and perspective to understand the meaning of a promise.

Be Flexible

When unusual situations arise, avoid sticking rigidly to your weaning plan. If your child is ill, for example, she may want to breastfeed more often for comfort. You can always go back to weaning after she's feeling better.

If These Strategies Don't Work

Even at the same age, some children will be more ready to wean than others. If your child becomes upset and cries or insists upon breastfeeding even when you try to distract or comfort her in others ways, this may mean that weaning is going too fast for her or that different strategies would be better. Other signs that weaning may be moving too fast are changes or regressions in behavior, such as stuttering, night-waking, an increase in clinginess, a new or increased fear of separation, biting (if she has never bitten before), stomach upsets, and constipation. Make weaning a positive experience for both you and your child by paying attention to your own inner voice and being sensitive to your child's cues.

Resources

Recommended Books, DVDs, and Websites

Books

Hale, T. 2012. *Medications and Mothers' Milk*, 15th ed. Amarillo, TX: Hale Publishing. Available from www.ibreastfeeding.com.

Mohrbacher, N. and K. Kendall-Tackett. 2010. *Breastfeeding Made Simple: Seven Natural Laws for Nursing Mothers*. 2nd ed. Oakland, CA: New Harbinger Publications.

Pantley, E. 2002. *The No-Cry Sleep Solution: Gentle Ways to Help Your Baby Sleep Through the Night*. New York: McGraw-Hill.

West, D. and L. Marasco. 2009. *The Breastfeeding Mother's Guide to Making More Milk*. New York: McGraw-Hill.

DVDs

Colson, S. 2011. *Biological Nurturing: Laid-Back Breastfeeding for Mothers.* Geddes Productions. Available from www.geddesproduction.com/breast-feeding-laid-back.php.

Websites

General Breastfeeding

Nancy Mohrbacher Breastfeeding Reporter: www.nancymohrbacher.com

KellyMom: www.kellymom.com

Breastfeeding USA: breastfeedingusa.org/breastfeeding-information

La Leche League International: www.llli.org/nb.html

Breastfeeding-Support Organizations

Breastfeeding USA: breastfeedingusa.org

La Leche League International: www.llli.org

United States Breastfeeding Committee: www.usbreastfeeding.org

International Lactation Consultant Association: www.ilca.org

Australian Breastfeeding Association: www.breastfeeding.asn.au

Academy of Breastfeeding Medicine: www.bfmed.org

Breastfeeding Positions

The Nurturing Project's laid-back breastfeeding video clip:
www.biologicalnurturing.com/video/bn3clip.html

Nancy Mohrbacher's resources on semi-reclined breastfeeding positions:
www.nancymohrbacher.com/blog/tag/laid-back-breastfeeding

Hand Expression

Amehhjelpen (a Norwegian mother-to-mother breastfeeding organization):
ammehjelpen.no/handmelking?id=907
(scroll down for the English version)

Stanford School of Medicine's "Hand Expression of Breastmilk" video clip:
newborns.stanford.edu/Breastfeeding/HandExpression.html

The Marmet Technique:
video.about.com/breastfeeding/Hand-Expression
-Technique.htm

Hands-On Pumping

Stanford School of Medicine's "Maximizing Milk Production with Hands-On Pumping" video clip:
newborns.stanford.edu/Breastfeeding/MaxProduction.html

Breastfeeding and Medications and Medical Procedures

Call the Infant Risk Center at 806-352-2519 Monday through Friday from 8 a.m. to 5 p.m. (CST) to speak to the experts.

Breastfeeding and Pumping Gear

Breast Pumps

Hygeia breast pumps: www.hygeiababy.com

Ameda breast pumps: www.ameda.com

Medela breast pumps: www.medelabreastfeedingus.com

At-Breast Supplementers

Lact-Aid Nursing Trainer: http.lact-aid.com

Medela Supplemental Nursing System (SNS):
www.nurturecenter.com/index.php?l=product_detail&
#0022;p=1255

Medela Starter SNS: Ask your hospital's lactation consultant where to find one in your area.

To read more about how to use these products, see:
www.lowmilksupply.org/abs.shtml.

Breast Shells

Ameda Breast Shell System:
http.amedadirect.com/ameda-duoshells-breastshells.html

Medela TheraShells:
www.toysrus.com/product/index.jsp?productId=2403242

Silicone Nipple Shields

Nipple shields come in different sizes and styles. For two
   common brands, see:
   www.amedadirect.com/ameda-nipple-shield.html
   www.medelabreastfeedingus.com/products/583/contact
   -nipple-shields

Soft Silicone Pump Inserts

Avent Isis Petal Massager:
   philipsparts.fox-international.com/PhilipsConsumerPart
   Detail.aspx?part=421333440070

Ameda Flexishield Areola Stimulator:
   www.ameda.com/ameda-products/spare-parts

Articles and Studies

From Introduction

Ip, S., M. Chung, G. Raman, P. Chew, N. Magula, D. DeVine, T.
   Trikalinos, and J. Lau. 2007. "Breastfeeding and Maternal
   and Infant Health Outcomes in Developed Countries."
   Evidence Report—Technology Assessment (Full Report)(153):
   1–186.

Bartick, M. and A. Reinhold. 2010. "The Burden of Suboptimal
   Breastfeeding in the United States: A Pediatric Cost
   Analysis." *Pediatrics* 125; e1048–e1056.

Stuebe, A. 2009. "The Risks of Not Breastfeeding for Mothers and Infants." *Reviews in Obstetrics & Gynecology* 2(4): 222–231, doi: 10.3909/riog0093.

From Chapter 1: Latching Struggles

Colson, S. D., J. H. Meek, et al. 2008. "Optimal Positions for the Release of Primitive Neonatal Reflexes Stimulating Breastfeeding." *Early Human Development* 84(7): 441–9.

From Chapters 3 and 4: Nipple Pain and Breast Pain

Eglash, A., M. B. Plane, and M. Mundt. 2006. "History, Physical and Laboratory Findings, and Clinical Outcomes of Lactating Women Treated with Antibiotics for Chronic Breast and/or Nipple Pain." *Journal of Human Lactation* 22(4): 429–432.

Livingstone, V. and L. J. Stringer. 1999. "The Treatment of Staphyloccocus Aureus–infected Sore Nipples: A Randomized Comparative Study." *Journal of Human Lactation* 15: 241–246.

From Chapter 5: Night Feedings

Blyton, D. M., C. E. Sullivan, and N. Edwards. 2002. "Lactation Is Associated with an Increase in Slow-Wave Sleep in Women." *Journal of Sleep Research* 11(4): 297–303.

Doan, T., A. Gardiner, C. L. Gay, and K. A. Lee. 2007. "Breastfeeding Increases Sleep Duration of New Parents." *Journal of Perinatal & Neonatal Nursing* 21(3): 200–206.

Kendall-Tackett, K., Z. Cong, and T. W. Hale. 2010. "Mother-Infant Sleep Locations and Nighttime Feeding Behaviors: U.S. Data from the Survey of Mothers' Sleep and Fatigue." *Clinical Lactation* 1(1): 27–31.

From Chapter 6: Pumping

Morton, J., J. Y. Hall, R. J. Wong, L. Thairu, W. E. Benitz, and W. D. Rhine. 2009. "Combining Hand Techniques with Electric Pumping Increases Milk Production in Mothers of Preterm Infants." *Journal of Perinatology* 29(11): 757–764.

From Chapter 7: Weaning

American Academy of Pediatrics section on breastfeeding. 2012. "Breastfeeding and the Use of Human Milk." *Pediatrics* 129(8): e827-e841.

Finding Skilled Breastfeeding Help

Finding skilled help can be tricky, in part because there are different breastfeeding credentials reflecting different levels of education and training. Some initials, such as CLC, CLE, CBE, CBC, and LE, are awarded after attending a brief training course, usually no more than one week long. A person with these initials may be helpful but may have limited skills and experience working one on one with breastfeeding mothers and babies.

The credential IBCLC indicates at the very least a basic competency in the field of lactation. These initials stand for *international board-certified lactation consultant*. To be awarded this credential, a person must pass an all-day certifying exam. And to qualify to take that exam, she must have a combination of formal education, breastfeeding education, and thousands of hours working one on one with breastfeeding mothers and babies. Here's how you can find an IBCLC:

- Click on "Find a Lactation Consultant" at www.ilca .org, the website of the International Lactation Consultant Association. Not all IBCLCs are members.

- Call your local hospital and ask to speak to the lactation consultant. Ask if she can help you or if she knows someone in your community who can.

- Contact a representative from a mother-to-mother breastfeeding organization, such as Breastfeeding USA, La Leche League, or the Australian Breastfeeding Association. These women are volunteers who have breastfed their own children and have at least a basic understanding of breastfeeding. Some are highly skilled and some are relatively inexperienced. Ideally, if your problem is more complicated than they can help with, or if you need to be seen and they are unable to do so, they will refer you to someone in your area who can provide the help you need.

Nancy Mohrbacher, IBCLC, FILCA, is the author and coauthor of several popular breastfeeding books, including *Breastfeeding Made Simple*, *Breastfeeding Answers Made Simple*, and *The Breastfeeding Answer Book*. She has helped thousands of breastfeeding families in the greater Chicago area, and in 2008 she was officially recognized by the International Lactation Consultant Association (ILCA).

Index

TUV

W

XYZ

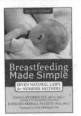
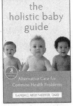

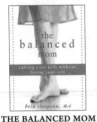
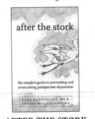
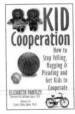